101 Careers in
Public Health

Beth Seltzer, MD, MPH, is a physician whose recent work has focused on using media as a tool for health education and behavior change. Dr. Seltzer is board-certified in public health and general preventive medicine. She attended medical school at Case Western Reserve University and completed her preventive medicine residency at Stony Brook University, with an MPH degree from Columbia University. Prior to her medical career, Dr. Seltzer was a documentary film producer, earning multiple awards for her work. More recently, she has been a writer and consultant for the Discovery Health and Discovery Channel television networks, developing content for educational television shows and interactive media directed at both physicians and general audiences.

101 Careers in Public Health

BETH SELTZER, MD, MPH

SPRINGER PUBLISHING COMPANY

NEW YORK

Springer Publishing Company, LLC
11 West 42nd Street
New York, NY 10036
www.springerpub.com

Acquisitions Editor: Jennifer Perillo
Cover Design: Mimi Flow
Composition: Newgen Imaging

ISBN: 978-0-8261-1768-7
E-ISBN: 978-0-8261-1769-4

12 13 / 5

The author and the publisher of this Work have made every effort to use sources believed to be reliable to provide information that is accurate and compatible at the time of publication. The publisher has no responsibility for the persistence or accuracy of URLs for external or third-party Internet Web sites referred to in this publication and does not guarantee that any content on such Web sites is, or will remain, accurate or appropriate.

Library of Congress Cataloging-in-Publication Data
  Seltzer, Beth.
  101 careers in public health / Beth Seltzer.
      p. cm.
  Includes index.
  ISBN: 978-0-8261-1768-7
      1. Public health—Vocational guidance. I. Title.   II. Title: One hundred and one careers in public health.
  RA440.9.S45 2010
  362.1023—dc22   2010022058

Special discounts on bulk quantities of our books are available to corporations, professional associations, pharmaceutical companies, health care organizations, and other qualifying groups. If you are interested in a custom book, including chapters from more than one of our titles, we can provide that service as well.

For details, please contact:
Special Sales Department, Springer Publishing Company, LLC
11 West 42nd Street, 15th Floor, New York, NY, 10036-8002
Phone: 877-687-7476 or 212-431-4370; Fax: 212-941-7842
Email: sales@springerpub.com

Printed in the United States of America by Hamilton Printing Company.

This book is dedicated to my parents,
Lynn and Robert Seltzer,
who have been right there with me
through my own 101 careers.

Contents

Preface

When I was in medical school, I was constantly frustrated by the number of people suffering from preventable diseases. Why was all the effort going into *treating* obesity-related diabetes instead of *preventing* it? We knew that a lot of our pediatric asthma patients would turn up in the emergency room again at some point after we discharged them from the hospital. Why weren't we figuring out why this kept happening, instead of accepting that these kids would be on a merry-go-round of asthma attacks and treatment? Teenagers with serious STDs, adults with untreated mental illness...the number of people who could have been helped by population-level efforts was astonishing to me.

I spent about three and a half years railing against all this, until one of my teachers finally introduced me to the world of public health. Here were the people who shared my frustration. Here was a whole world of doctors, nurses, social workers, research scientists, administrators, and activists trying to get those kids off the asthma merry-go-round, trying to shift the way America eats and convince us to ramp up our exercise levels to halt the epidemic of diabetes, and working with teenagers to encourage safer sexual practices and slow the spread of STDs.

I've since completed my medical residency and become board-certified in preventive medicine, a specialty with a focus on public health. My fellow "prev med" physicians are an extraordinary group of people, and I think most of us are delighted to have found our way here. As I was interviewing people for this book—health inspectors, civil engineers, pharmacists, and a range of other experts—every single one of them shared their excitement about being part of public health.

I'm delighted that you've picked up this book, and I hope it will inspire you to pursue a career in public health. It is a great field to be in.

Welcome. I hope you'll love it here as much as I do.

—*Beth Seltzer, MD, MPH*

Acknowledgments

A heartfelt thank you to the extraordinarily generous people who contributed their time, wisdom, and experience to this book. Much of what you'll learn here comes from them. Any errors are entirely mine.

Thank-you to all the people who shared their stories for the public health profiles. Many of you agreed to participate with just a brief introduction to the project, because you wanted to help students and career-changers learn about your job. Your kindness made working on this book an absolute joy.

Thanks also to everyone who helped me create the list of careers, taught me what people in each job actually do all day, checked my descriptions to make sure they rang true, responded to a request for information, or connected me with another resource. I'll try to name everyone here; please forgive me if I've left you out, and know that I very much appreciate your contribution.

Much gratitude to: Pat McConnan, Wanda Manson, Beth Lamanna, Madelaine Fletcher, Candace McCall, Julie Wu, Michael Zwick, Chet Moore, Liz Garman, Aletha Maybank, James Gaudino, Catherine Hayes, Keith Hauret, Mary Anne Bright, Linda Bailey, Chris Anderson, Vickie Wightman, Andrea Circe, Jim Lando, Sheree Williams, Jodee Denneson, Steve Blessing, Leslie Sandler, Kathy Jacobitz, Elizabeth Scharman, Carolyn Barth, Stephen Cina, Stephanie Birch, Robert Burke, Rita Ruel, Julian Kesner, Carol Odnoha, Kate Corona, Susan Johnson, Andrea Gatewood, Douglas Steinke, Rebecca Garner, Kate Migliaccio, Karen Mahoney, Gary Schnabel, Robert Hart, Anne Wright, Vonni Kallemeyn, Ryan Benefield, Jim Kubat, James Tacci, David Hicks, Kelly Classic, Cynthia Jones, Debbie Gilley, Dilcia Granville, Christopher Kelly, Jill Cruickshank, Julie Stallcup, Jennifer McEntire, Martin Lo, Michael Herndon, Wes Long, Stephanie Berger, Irwin Redlener, Patricia Thomas, Nedra Weinreich, John Curtis, Martin Snyder, Paula Kun, Becky Smith, Ephraim Shapiro, Anita Nelson, Steve Smothers, Deb Schnellman,

Jeanne Saunders, Theresa Spinner, Reg Hutchinson, Cindy Sweigert, R. Gerald ("Bobby") Smith, Mark Casanova, Bernadette Burden, Karen White, Sherry Glied, Rachael Wojnowicz, Chuck Young, Eric Wedum, James Schuttinga, Rina Lieberman, Yair Goldstein, Ben Meier, Gene Matthews, Bev Thomas, Jo Ann Saringer, Tyrone Butler, Melissa Lewis, John Porter, Dorothy Lane, Philip Baten, Patti Jo Baber, Laurie Shroyer, Vikas Tandon, Karen Greenwood, Jacqueline Neilsen, Deanna Kramer, John Skendall, Kelly Romero, Christine Clayton, Jody Devoll, Laura Crawford, Ashgar Rastegar, Jennifer Johnsen, Tonia Poteat, Carolyn Hart, Bill Kaizer, and Tanya Cobbs Leslie. Special thanks to George Johns, Tracey Lynn, Kathleen Scanlin, James Horan, Carmit Keddem, Don Griffin, and Julia Goodall.

Thank you to my friends who made connections for me or reviewed parts of the manuscript, including Esther Sitrin, Kevin Hogan, Christy English, Alisa Roost, Katey Coffing, Shannah Whithaus, and Noeleen Walder; to Diana Goodwin, for always being there when I need her; and to everyone else who put up with me while I was working on this project. Sincere appreciation, too, to Professor Steven Jonas at Stony Brook University, for believing I could do this in the first place.

And finally, thanks to Jennifer Perillo at Springer Publishing Company, who has not only made my writing better, but also demonstrated more patience than anyone has a right to expect.

101 Careers in Public Health

Introduction to Public Health

1 What Is Public Health?

Public health professionals sometimes joke that nobody understands what they do—until something goes wrong. We tend to take it for granted that the water from our kitchen faucets is safe to drink. We rarely worry about tuberculosis, measles, or diphtheria. We assume that medicine we buy from the local pharmacy will make us better, not make us ill. But when dozens of people are sickened at a restaurant or if there is an outbreak of a deadly illness, *then* everyone asks why the health department hasn't been doing its job!

Public health is the discipline that aims to keep our population safe from illness. Unlike a doctor who treats individual patients (usually once they are already sick), the public health expert considers health from the perspective of entire communities, neighborhoods, cities, and states. Public health even addresses disease prevention and health promotion on a national and global scale.

HISTORY OF PUBLIC HEALTH

Public health measures have been around for centuries. Excavation of a 4,000-year-old city in India revealed covered sewers to carry waste away from people's homes. In Rome about 2,000 years ago, a system of aqueducts brought fresh water to the city. Legend has it that 2,500 years ago, a Greek emperor ended a malaria epidemic by changing the course of two rivers, making a marshy region less hospitable to mosquitoes.

The idea of quarantining people who were contagious became prominent in the Middle Ages. To combat leprosy, Church leaders decided to separate people with leprosy from the rest of society, making life very difficult for those patients, but probably saving many healthy citizens from contracting the disease. Similar measures were used when the Black Plague hit.

Of course, people haven't always understood disease the way we do today. Some misunderstandings actually led to effective public health efforts—the idea that disease was caused by "bad air" eventually led to improvements in sanitation. But confusion about how diseases spread also led to less successful approaches. In Europe in the 1800s, government officials tried to stop the spread of cholera by quarantining people who were ill, destroying their belongings, and burying the dead immediately and away from highly populated areas. But none of these activities actually stopped cholera epidemics.

The roots of modern epidemiology, one of the most important sciences in public health today, are widely thought to lie in work that was done around that time. Epidemiology is the study of how diseases occur within populations and how they can be controlled. Although no one knew exactly what caused cholera, John Snow, a doctor practicing in London, realized that the key to stopping outbreaks lay in figuring out how cholera was being transmitted. Instead of focusing on the disease in individual patients, he looked for patterns in where and when cases of cholera occurred. His investigation led to the discovery that outbreaks were linked to contaminated water, and could be halted by providing a clean water supply. Snow wasn't the only one who attempted to use epidemiologic methods, but his story is among the most well known. It took years for his ideas to be accepted, but approaches similar to his are now widely considered to be at the heart of modern public health.

THE ROLE OF PUBLIC HEALTH TODAY

Today, public health is far more than providing clean water, maintaining sanitation, and controlling the spread of contagious diseases. The field has expanded to include prevention of chronic diseases and cancer, the control of conditions that are linked to disease, like obesity, and attention to mental health. There are public health experts studying disparities in levels of disease among different racial and ethnic groups, and trying to bring everyone up to the same degree of health. Public health topics also include infant mortality, access to dental care, the prevention of drug and alcohol abuse, and even seat belt and helmet laws. Public health techniques are used to promote workplace safety and reduce on-the-job injuries. Public health can even include clinics and other services to individuals, when those services are offered in the context of trying to raise the health of a community or group.

In fact, the field of public health has become so broad that even the people who practice it have trouble defining exactly what public health means today. In general, what public health efforts have in common is a focus on promoting health at the population level, instead of focusing on the individual interactions between doctor and patient. The Institute of Medicine offered a definition in their 1988 report *The Future of Public Health*. The report specified the mission of public health as "fulfilling society's interest in assuring conditions in which people can be healthy." It also identified three core functions:

- **Assessment.** Public health agencies should collect and analyze information about the health of the communities they serve.
- **Policy Development.** Agencies should promote the use of sound science and act as leaders in the development of comprehensive public health policies.
- **Assurance.** Agencies should assure the provision of services necessary to meet public health goals.

Federal agencies and public health organizations got together a few years later and expanded the definition with the following list of 10 essential public health services:

1. **Monitor** health status to identify community health problems.
2. **Diagnose and investigate** health problems and health hazards in the community.
3. **Inform, educate, and empower** people about health issues.
4. **Mobilize** community partnerships to identify and solve health problems.
5. **Develop** policies and plans that support individual and community health efforts.
6. **Enforce** laws and regulations that protect health and ensure safety.

7. **Link** people to needed personal health services and assure the provision of health care when otherwise unavailable.
8. **Assure** a competent public health and personal health care workforce.
9. **Evaluate** effectiveness, accessibility, and quality of personal and population-based health services.
10. **Research** for new insights and innovative solutions to health problems.

Monitoring, Diagnosis, and Investigation

Monitoring is at the root of many public health efforts. If we don't know what patterns of disease are occurring, we can't create rational programs to address those diseases. In the United States, certain contagious diseases are considered "reportable," which means that doctors or laboratories must alert health officials whenever a case is discovered. If there is an unusually high number of cases, public health experts swing into action to find out why. Public health agencies also monitor diabetes, heart disease, cancer, birth defects, certain types of injuries, and other serious medical problems. A sudden increase in disease, especially if it's in a single location, can signal an immediate problem to be addressed. Even a gradual, widespread change can expose the need for improved health measures on a local or national scale.

Disease Prevention and Health Promotion

Once a problem (such as infectious disease, chronic disease, or injury) has been identified, public health experts use a wide range of methods to try to prevent it from happening. Water treatment plants, free clinics to treat and prevent the spread of sexually transmitted infections, and ad campaigns promoting exercise are all examples of disease prevention efforts. So are programs to reduce pollution and to encourage stores to stock more healthful foods. From low-cost vaccinations for children to national recommendations for exercise, the active prevention of disease and promotion of health are enormous parts of modern public health activities.

Research

The best public health efforts are based on sound research. At schools of public health, government agencies, and nonprofit organizations, scientists work on finding the best approaches to maintaining and improving health on a population level. Researchers are looking at how our environment affects our health. They are examining why certain populations seem to have consistently better health outcomes than others. They are working on ways to evaluate existing public health programs to see what works and where our tax dollars should be spent. And they are studying public health from many other angles, from the impact of personal choices to the effects of national policy.

Policy

Many public health programs and services are provided by local, state, and federal government agencies. These efforts are created and controlled by laws and regulations. Even nonprofit organizations operate according to overarching policies. A good policy provides for sound, science-based monitoring and prevention and may also support necessary research. But even policies that come from the best intentions can have unintended consequences. There are public health experts who study the outcomes of past policies, examine the impact of current ones, and advise legislators and other policymakers on how to make good choices for the future.

Health Services Research

Health services research is sometimes considered a separate category from public health, but many public health experts consider it a part of the continuum. Health services research looks at how health care is delivered, including the effects of billing and financial structures; the organization of hospitals, insurance companies, and medical practices; the use of health technologies; and the behavior of individuals. Researchers in this area look at patient outcomes, access to care, how people utilize doctors and hospitals, and how health care differs for different populations. The information they collect can be used by doctors, patients, hospitals, insurance companies, policymakers, and others, and the overall goal—at least from the public health perspective—is to improve health care for all.

Direct Service

There are many public health efforts that incorporate direct patient care. There are local and national hotlines to help people quit smoking, provide assistance in cases of accidental poisoning, and direct victims of domestic violence to services. Emergency medical services use a public health perspective, aiming not only to match their services to community needs but also standing ready to serve in case of disaster or attack. Many members of the U.S. Public Health Service Commissioned Corps are assigned to the Indian Health Service (IHS), which provides comprehensive health services to American Indians and Alaska Natives.

REFERENCES

Centers for Disease Control and Prevention. National Public Health Performance Standards Program. *Ten essential public health services.* Retrieved from http://www.cdc.gov/od/ocphp/nphpsp/EssentialPHServices.htm. Accessed on March 23, 2010.

Institute of Medicine Committee for the Study of the Future of Public Health. (1988). *The future of public health.* Washington, DC: National Academies Press.

Porter, D. (1999). Health, civilization, and the state: A history of public health from ancient to modern times. New York: Routledge.

Rosen, G. (1958). *A history of public health.* New York: MD Publications, Inc.

2 | Education in Public Health

There are many roads to a career in public health, and it is common to meet people who started out in different careers entirely. Some began as hospital nurses or physicians in clinical practice; others were lawyers, teachers, or even journalists. For many public health jobs, the Master of Public Health (MPH) degree is considered the most appropriate, but there are also jobs for which additional credentials—or entirely different ones—are essential.

BACHELOR'S DEGREES IN PUBLIC HEALTH

Some schools offer a bachelor of science in public health degree. This degree is designed to give students a basic grounding in public health issues and methods. There are also bachelor's degrees available in environmental health, health promotion, community health sciences, and other related majors. For some public health jobs, this level of education is appropriate. Many people working in public health today actually majored in other fields, however, and for many jobs a broader education is useful.

For students who plan to pursue an MPH, the Association of Schools of Public Health (ASPH) notes that many different majors can be good foundations. Sociology, psychology, or anthropology can be useful majors for those interested in behavioral science or health education; biology or chemistry for those interested in environmental health; and biology or one of the social sciences for those who lean toward maternal and child health issues.

MASTER'S OF PUBLIC HEALTH DEGREES

People who have been in public health for many years often don't have MPH degrees, but it seems this degree is becoming more expected for certain positions. MPH programs offer a sound background in core public health topics, including epidemiology, biostatistics, environmental health, health policy and management, and social and behavioral sciences. The educational requirements include coursework, a practical experience or internship in a public health setting, and a final thesis, examination, or other demonstration of comprehensive knowledge and the ability to apply it. Some programs offer a generalist degree, but it is common for schools to require students to choose an area of concentration. In addition to the core topics, various schools offer concentrations such as global health, population sciences, community health, and program management.

Different schools of public health can be quite different in their offerings, priorities, and requirements, so it is important to pay attention to which school you choose. Most MPH programs last for 2 years, although some are designed to be completed in a shorter time.

DOCTOR'S OF PUBLIC HEALTH DEGREES

The Doctor of Public Health (DrPH) degree is for people with an interest in public health leadership, or a desire for deeper knowledge than an MPH program can provide. It is generally considered a degree for those who intend to be leaders in research programs, policymaking, or public health practice. It requires several years of study, an original research project, and a lengthy written dissertation. A DrPH can serve as preparation for a research career, but a PhD with a narrower focus is often more appropriate for someone interested primarily in conducting research and pursuing an academic career.

COMBINED DEGREE PROGRAMS

Many schools offer programs combining the MPH with another degree, such as nursing, medicine, law, or social work. These programs vary in focus, so it is important to explore the coursework and requirements.

OTHER MASTER'S DEGREES

A number of other master's degrees, besides the MPH, are common among people working in public health. For someone interested in administration—managing a bureau within a state health department, for example—a Master's of Public Administration (MPA) can be very helpful. A Master's of Public Policy (MPP) focuses on policy analysis, design, and implementation. There is also a Master of Science in Public Health degree, with an emphasis on research. Some public health professionals find that a Master's of Business Administration (MBA) is useful, either to help them understand how health-related businesses function, or to give them perspective on management issues.

ENGINEERING DEGREES

For those people who handle the nuts and bolts of our water system, design and manage sewer systems, and make sure landfills are properly constructed, a background in engineering is key. These people often don't have degrees in "public health" at all—instead, they have degrees in civil or environmental engineering. There are bachelor's degrees, master's degrees, and PhDs available in these fields. The level of education needed depends on the specific job responsibilities.

CERTIFICATIONS AND OTHER TRAINING

Some public health jobs require other types of training, and some require state licensure. The inspectors who keep an eye on the use of dangerous radioactive materials, for example, receive extensive training on the job. The people who answer the phone at the poison control hotline must pass a test sponsored by a national organization. The National Board of

Public Health Examiners (NBPHE) also recently began offering a voluntary public health certification examination; you can find out more at www.nbphe.org. As you read through this book, you'll see examples of training and certifications required for specific jobs.

FINDING A SCHOOL OF PUBLIC HEALTH

Schools of public health are located within universities throughout the United States. A list of accredited schools is available through the ASPH Web site at www.asph.org. This site also includes information about requirements for public health degrees and some advice about careers.

3   Finding Jobs in Public Health

There are many different ways to join the ranks of people working in public health. As you'll learn from the people who shared their stories for this book, it is quite common for people to have reached their current jobs through roundabout paths. Here's a basic outline of the different ways to begin a career in public health.

TRADITIONAL PATHWAYS

Some people go to school, earn a Master of Public Health (MPH) or another degree, and immediately apply for a job that matches the focus of their studies. Many MPH students are hired to work at places where they interned. Others use the network of people they meet during their studies to find job openings and get recommendations. Some simply answer an ad. Good Web sites for public health job postings include:

- Publichealthjobs.net, a job board provided by the Association of Schools of Public Health
- APHA's Career Development Center, careers.apha.org/careerdev, which offers job listings, career tips, career coaching, and more
- USAJOBS.gov, the U.S. government's job board for opportunities at federal agencies

■ Idealist.org, a job board for nonprofit organizations including groups concerned with public health

For people interested in jobs with the federal government, there are several opportunities for fellowships and training programs. Not all of these are well known, even among people currently working in public health. Opportunities include:

■ **Epidemic Intelligence Service (EIS).** Many of the top people in public health agencies began their careers in EIS. EIS is a 2-year, postgraduate training program—complete with a livable salary—that combines classroom learning and on-the-job training in applied epidemiology. The program is primarily intended for people with doctoral-level degrees (including MDs, PhDs, dentists, and veterinarians), but people with MPHs can also be accepted. Participants learn to investigate disease outbreaks and other potential public health problems, analyze patterns of illness and injury, and design a public health surveillance system.

■ **Department of Health and Human Services (HHS) Emerging Leaders Program (ELP).** The divisions of HHS include the Food and Drug Administration, the National Institutes of Health, the Centers for Disease Control and Prevention (CDC), and other agencies concerned with public health. ELP is a competitive 2-year "internship" that includes a salary and planned promotions. Interns rotate through different departments within HHS and receive mentoring from senior executives. Applicants must have a relevant master's degree, meet certain other educational requirements, or have at least a year of relevant, specialized experience.

■ **Presidential Management Fellows (PMF) Program.** This prestigious program is intended to attract graduate students from various disciplines into federal service, as future leaders in the management of public policies and programs. Becoming a fellow in this 2-year paid program requires nomination by a dean, director, or chairperson of one's graduate academic program. The CDC is among the agencies that offer these fellowships.

■ **Public Health Prevention Service (PHPS).** PHPS is a fellowship program at the CDC for people with MPH degrees or with management-related degrees plus academic work related to public health. Applicants must also have 1 year of public health work experience. The 3-year program is intended to train future leaders in public health. There is also a Public Health Apprenticeship program, a 2-year fellowship for recent college graduates interested in public health careers.

There is more information about fellowships and training programs at CDC's public health training opportunities Web site, www.cdc.gov/phtrain/training_programs.html.

Another opportunity is the U.S. Public Health Service (USPHS) Commissioned Corps. The Commissioned Corps is one of our seven uniformed services—along with the Army, Navy, Air Force, Marines, Coast Guard, and National Oceanic and Atmospheric Administration Commissioned Corps. The doctors, dentists, nurses, pharmacists, engineers, and others in the USPSH Commissioned Corps wear uniforms and have military-style rank. They have opportunities to serve in government agencies throughout the United States and even overseas.

There are also public health jobs in the U.S. military, both for service members and for civilians. Many of the jobs in this book have counterparts in the armed services.

GETTING IN THE BACK DOOR

Many people, even those with long careers in public health, still express surprise that they "ended up" in this field. Many found their first job through volunteering. A volunteer experience with a nonprofit organization can give you a first-hand look at the needs of communities and provide training in health education, monitoring, and even program design, coordination, and evaluation. It can also introduce you to potential mentors and a network of people who are aware of your abilities and interests. Volunteering can lead to a job with that organization or another one with similar goals. And, since some employers will accept experience in lieu of a public health degree, a volunteering experience can actually launch a career.

Organizations and associations for public health professionals can also provide networking opportunities. Local meetings and national conferences are good places to meet people who are doing the work you're interested in, and they'll usually be happy to talk with you. You might meet someone who knows of just the job for a person with your skills.

You might also learn about a fellowship or other paid training program that is a good match for your background and your goals.

COMBINING PUBLIC HEALTH WITH ANOTHER CAREER

Social workers, nurses, dentists, and doctors can sometimes combine public health work with a clinical career, working part-time for a health department or community clinic. Some advertising professionals donate a portion of their time to ad campaigns that promote good health instead of selling products. Even executives at for-profit corporations can get involved in "corporate responsibility" programs that promote health on a population scale.

PROFESSIONAL ASSOCIATIONS

Throughout this book, you'll read about professional associations and organizations associated with specific jobs and careers. One of the best and most comprehensive resources for people interested in public health work is APHA. APHA's annual meeting attracts thousands of people from a wide range of careers. APHA has low-cost membership options and discounts on annual meeting registration for students and "consumer members" (people not currently working in public health). You can learn more about APHA at www.apha.org.

FEDERAL GOVERNMENT AGENCIES

The U.S. Department of Health and Human Services (HHS) is the principal federal agency tasked with protecting the public's health and providing certain social services. It incorporates multiple agencies, each of which has at least some programs that address public health issues.

- **Administration for Children and Families (ACF).** ACF focuses on the economic and social well-being of families, children, individuals, and communities.
- **Administration on Aging (AoA).** AoA's mission is to develop a system of home-based and community-based services to help the elderly maintain their independence and their health.

- **Agency for Health Care Research and Quality (AHRQ).** AHRQ supports research on health care quality, costs, and outcomes, as well as efforts to improve quality, cost-effectiveness, and access to care.
- **Agency for Toxic Substances and Disease Registry (ATSDR).** ATSDR's focus is the prevention of diseases related to toxic substances and exposures to substances that can be harmful.
- **CDC.** CDC's efforts include monitoring, research, programs, services, and policy development related to health promotion, disease prevention, prevention of injury and disability, and preparedness for new health threats.
- **Centers for Medicare & Medicaid Services (CMS).** CMS handles the administration of Medicare and, on the federal level, of Medicaid and the Children's Health Insurance Program.
- **Food and Drug Administration (FDA).** FDA is tasked with assuring the safety, effectiveness, and security of prescription medications, over-the-counter drugs, and certain other health-related products, as well as cosmetics, tobacco, and certain aspects of our food supply.
- **Health Resources and Services Administration (HRSA).** HRSA's mission is to improve access to health care, with a focus on people who are uninsured, isolated or medically vulnerable.
- **Indian Health Service (IHS).** IHS provides personal and public health services to American Indians and Alaska Natives, with the goal of maximizing these populations' physical, mental, social, and spiritual health.
- **National Institutes of Health (NIH).** The focus of work at NIH is the practice and support of medical research.
- **Office of Inspector General (OIG).** OIG keeps an eye on HHS programs, makes sure they are properly managed, and aims to ensure the health and welfare of program beneficiaries.
- **Substance Abuse and Mental Health Services Administration (SAMHSA).** SAMHSA focuses on mental health issues, and its mission is to build resilience and facilitate recovery.

Several other federal agencies have roles in protecting and enhancing the public's health. Public health-oriented programs and practices can be found at agencies including:

- The U.S. Department of Agriculture (USDA)
- The Environmental Protection Agency (EPA)

- The Consumer Product Safety Commission (CPSC)
- The U.S. Department of Labor's Occupational Safety and Health Administration (OSHA)

STATE AND LOCAL AGENCIES

State, county, and city health departments have multiple divisions that add to federal efforts and take additional steps to meet local needs. The exact structure of state and local health services varies from place to place, but there is an enormous range of opportunities at these levels for professionals pursuing careers in public health. Visit the Web sites of your state and city or county health departments to see the roles they play in water quality, environmental health, maternal and child health, nutrition, patient safety, and more.

Public Health Careers

4 Infectious Disease

In spite of advances in clinical medicine, infectious disease remains an important public health concern. Even with widespread immunization, outbreaks of diseases like measles and mumps continue to occur. New infectious agents are constantly being discovered. The ease of international travel means that infectious agents are easily carried from one part of the world to another. The development of resistance to antibiotics and antiviral medications presents new challenges. In some parts of the world, limited access to medicine means that even curable infections can be devastating.

Public health efforts to combat infectious diseases include collecting data about the symptoms patients report and the diagnoses they receive, watching for unusual cases, and investigating outbreaks. When an outbreak or epidemic occurs, public health officials take action to inform the public, educate physicians, and develop policies and systems to contain the infection. There are also policies and programs to keep known infectious agents under control, so that outbreaks are less likely to happen.

This chapter will introduce you to some of the careers that involve the control of infectious diseases. To learn about others, also see behavioral scientist, medical epidemiologist, employee health nurse, corporate medical director, health inspector, consumer safety officer, and health educator. The CDC Web site (www.cdc.gov) is a great resource for an introduction to infection control and public health.

EPIDEMIOLOGIST

Job Description

Epidemiologists are scientists who study the causes of disease in populations, how diseases spread, and what puts people at risk. They look at issues such as which populations are most affected, what the people who are infected have in common, and whether people who get sick are more likely to have certain risk factors than those who remain healthy. Most epidemiologists' work involves numbers and statistics; they figure out what information should be gathered, how it should be analyzed, and how it can be used. Sometimes they help explain study results to policymakers, the media, and the public. Some epidemiologists also work on ways to prevent disease.

Epidemiologists can study multiple types of diseases, or they can specialize—in infectious diseases, chronic diseases, or other topics such as genetic disorders, workplace injuries, violence or accidents, or how the environment influences people's health. An epidemiologist's job can be very creative and exciting, such as tracking a dangerous new virus. The work can also be more solitary, such as monitoring how many people test positive for tuberculosis (TB) each year. The job is usually office-based and involves a lot of computer time.

Education and Certification

Most epidemiologists have at least a master's degree, generally an MPH, with a specific focus on epidemiology. For upper-level positions, a doctorate is usually needed—but a fulfilling career is possible with only master's degree. Some epidemiologists have a background in medicine or nursing, combined with a degree, coursework, or other training in epidemiology. (See "Medical Epidemiologist" to learn more.)

Core Competencies and Skills

- Tendency to think logically and analytically
- Interest in solving challenging research problems
- Ability to work both individually and collaboratively
- Desire to continue learning about new topics and new techniques
- Strong background in math and statistics
- Knowledge of how to use statistics programs and databases

■ Ability to explain statistics, study design, and study results to people with different educational backgrounds

Compensation

Nationwide, the median salary for an epidemiologist is about $61,000, with most earning between $40,000 and $93,000, although senior-level epidemiologists can earn more. Epidemiologists with doctoral degrees usually start at higher salaries, and have a higher earning potential than those with master's degrees.

Workplaces

Many epidemiologists work for government agencies, such as the CDC, the National Cancer Institute, and city, state, and local health departments. Epidemiologists can also be found at universities, in hospitals, at consulting firms, and in other organizations or companies that do work related to health.

Employment Outlook

National data suggest that most states are facing a shortage of qualified epidemiologists. The Council of State and Territorial Epidemiologists also estimates that a larger workforce is needed to carry out all essential public health services. If budgets allow, an ongoing expansion in the field of applied epidemiology—with increasing interest in chronic disease, maternal and child health, substance abuse, and other health care issues—may create new jobs. Existing jobs tend to be relatively stable in difficult economic times.

For Further Information

■ Council of State and Territorial Epidemiologists (CSTE)
  www.cste.org
■ American College of Epidemiology (ACE)
  www.acepidemiology.org
■ American Public Health Association—Epidemiology section
  http://www.apha.org/membergroups/sections/aphasections/
  epidemiology/
■ The Society for Healthcare Epidemiology of America (SHEA)
  www.shea-online.org

PUBLIC HEALTH PROFILE: Epidemiologist
Orion McCotter, MPH

Border Infectious Disease Surveillance Epidemiologist
Arizona Department of Health Services, Tucson, AZ

Describe the sort of work you do.

My role at the Arizona Department of Health Services is part of the Border Infectious Disease Surveillance program (BIDS). BIDS was created to survey infectious disease along the US-Mexico border. The participants include local, state, federal, and international public health agencies from each country. My work involves surveillance for infectious diseases near the border between Arizona and Sonora, Mexico. I monitor the occurrence of diseases and watch for new patterns of infection that could signal an outbreak or epidemic.

What is a typical day like at your job?

The daily routine changes constantly depending on what is currently a public heath threat. For example, we are in the midst of an influenza pandemic. I have been conducting analyses of emergency room patients that have flu-like symptoms, and trying to determine the proportion of the disease that is confirmed by laboratory tests. When I get results, I notify the hospital, the local health department, and the state epidemiologist. I then write an Arizona BIDS report to share the information with hospitals and public health offices in my region. I am able to perform active surveillance for different infectious diseases in a similar way.

I am often in the field, at clinic or hospital sites, to train health care staff on surveillance methods. I travel to meet with epidemiologists and public health officials. There are also regular phone conferences with colleagues.

What education or training do you have? Is it typical for your job?

I have a BS in health education with a community emphasis, focused on disease prevention and health promotion. I have an MPH with a primary concentration in epidemiology and a secondary concentration in health policy. It took a little extra time to do that secondary

Continued

concentration, but it's been really valuable. It helps me to understand how to translate its findings into policies or interventions that will benefit the public. Many people who do a job like mine would have an MPH with a focus on epidemiology. Some of the people I work with have PhDs, and medical epidemiologists have MDs.

What path did you take to get to the job you are in today?

I discovered public health during my second year at college. I wanted to do something that would help people. Some time after college, I went back to school and I took a class at the public health college. Through that class, I worked with the local health department to do a community assessment of childhood injury. That's when I rediscovered public health and decided to go into the MPH program. I started working for the state as an independent contractor, and eventually I was able to move into my current position.

Where might you go from here, if you wanted to advance your career?

Someone in my job might advance within the health department in several ways. A first step might be to become a program manager. Program managers may be offered promotion to manage an entire section or bureau. Many people continue with higher education in order to advance their careers. I am interested in pursuing a PhD in epidemiology, or potentially a clinical degree.

What is the worst or most challenging part of your job?

Sometimes things don't move at the speed that I would like. Within any agency, there are many layers of approval and review before things are able to move forward. Just because I think a project is ready to go, does not mean it is going to start moving yet.

What is the best part?

I enjoy the vast network of people that I get to work with: laboratory directors, emergency room physicians, infection control practitioners,

Continued

infectious disease physicians, and epidemiologists. I also collaborate with colleagues from the University of Arizona College of Medicine and College of Public Health.

What advice do you have for someone who is interested in your career?

APHA and CSTE are great organizations for networking, and they welcome students. Find out about people's careers and what they typically do. The role of a local epidemiologist is different from a state epidemiologist, and different from a federal job.

MEDICAL OFFICER

Job Description

"Medical officers" are physicians who provide medical expertise for city, state, or federal agencies. Medical officers offer specialized knowledge of disease and treatment that can be essential to making good public health decisions. A medical officer's specific job can include doing direct medical care as part of a government program, but often it involves big-picture work such as developing guidelines and policies, giving advice about the safety of new technologies and products, conducting research on disease prevention and control, making decisions about government grants, or providing guidance for epidemiologic surveillance.

In infectious disease control, there are medical officers who study how infections spread, and then help create recommendations to prevent or control outbreaks. Some help design and carry out disease control programs. Other jobs include helping evaluate antibiotics or other products used to battle infectious disease, participating in infectious disease surveillance and the interpretation of epidemiologic data, and carrying out research. There are medical officers not just in infectious disease control but in many areas of public health, including maternal and child health, chronic disease control, injury prevention, and global health.

Medical officers often enjoy reasonable work hours in comfortable surroundings, although some jobs include emergency response after hours. (For more opportunities for physicians in public health, see medical epidemiologist, medical officer/drug safety, and physician/global health.)

Education and Certification

A medical officer must have an MD or Doctor of Osteopathic Medicine (DO) degree and usually must be licensed to practice medicine. Requirements regarding residency training and other preparation vary according to the needs of each job. For some jobs, earning an MPH or becoming board-certified in preventive medicine can make a candidate more competitive. For others, expertise in a relevant clinical specialty is essential.

Core Competencies and Skills

- Good critical thinking skills
- Ability to think flexibly
- Interest in continuing to learn new information and skills
- Willingness to follow government regulations and cope with red tape
- At least a basic grounding in epidemiology and biostatistics
- Understanding of relevant public health regulations and the structure of health-related agencies
- Medical knowledge appropriate to the specific job

Compensation

Medical officers are usually paid well, although not in keeping with the salaries of surgeons or other highly paid specialists. Typical salaries with the federal government range from about $90,000 to about $150,000. Federal workers also receive generous benefits packages.

Workplaces

The agencies within HHS employ a large number of medical officers to do work related to public health. In addition to jobs at federal government agencies, there are similar opportunities with state and local health departments, international agencies, and other organizations, although the job title may be different. (The term "medical officer" is also used in other contexts that do not necessarily have to do with public health.)

Employment Outlook

Several states report a shortage of public health physicians or expect a shortage in the near future. Most health departments have jobs that are designated specifically for physicians, and at any given moment there are many listings for medical officers on the Web site USAJOBS.gov. Finding the job you want can take time, but public health doctors can enjoy broad opportunities for advancement and for lateral moves once they have entered the system. The U.S. Public Health Service Commissioned Corps can also provide steady employment and a long-term career.

For Further Information

■ There is no single organization for public health medical officers, but the American College of Preventive Medicine (ACPM) (www.acpm. org) is a good resource.

PUBLIC HEALTH PROFILE: Medical Officer
George Pourakis, MD, MPH
Medical Officer
Centers for Disease Control and Prevention, Atlanta, GA

Describe the sort of work you do.

I'm part of a team addressing community measures to prevent the spread of novel H1N1 influenza, the so-called "swine flu" that was first detected in 2009. Visit the CDC Web site and go to www.cdc. gov/h1n1flu/guidance. My team creates the guidance documents. We provide recommendations for prevention in various community settings. We're working on guidance for mass gatherings like business conferences, and next we'll be doing one for homeless shelters. Our recommendations are not binding in terms of law, but people throughout the country look at them to see what they should do.

What is a typical day like at your job?

I'm involved in both gathering information for guidance documents and the actual writing. I spend a fair amount of time reviewing prior guidance

Continued

documents to identify what aspects are relevant to the new setting I'm writing about. Then, I talk with appropriate subject matter experts. I also search the medical literature to find the best possible evidence about preventing the spread of this strain of influenza and the flu in general. I send our drafts out to various stakeholders, including state and local health officials and professional organizations. They send comments back, and then I review the comments and figure out how to incorporate them. I also respond to questions about the documents.

What education or training do you have? Is it typical for your job?

I have an MD and an MPH. My medical specialty is public health and general preventive medicine. I don't know that an MD is essential for this particular job, but a clinical background is an asset. You have to understand the principles of disease transmission and prevention. Public health training is essential for this work.

What path did you take to get to the job you are in today?

I did a year of an anesthesiology residency, but I realized I wanted my work to have a broader impact. I switched to preventive medicine, which has a strong focus on public health. During that residency, I did an internship with ACPM in Washington, D.C. Through contacts I made, I was able to intern with the Committee on Oversight and Government Reform in the U.S. House of Representatives. I worked on briefings and hearings dealing with H1N1 vaccine manufacturing, distribution, and safety.

After my residency training, I submitted my resume on the USAjobs.gov Web site. I was invited to a CDC job fair in Atlanta. They were recruiting people to work on issues surrounding H1N1, and I had the experience they were looking for.

Where might you go from here, if you wanted to advance your career?

I'm interested in the impact that legislation has on public health. So I'm hoping that the work I'm doing now, and my connections at the

Continued

CDC and elsewhere, will eventually lead to a role focusing more on health policy. For someone who's interested in infectious disease, specifically, the best next step would probably be to do the Epidemic Intelligence Service program and become a medical epidemiologist. Having done EIS can help you get your foot in the door in lots of areas.

What is the worst or most challenging part of your job?

When you're at a federal agency, you're in the spotlight. You're subject to the scrutiny of everyone—the public, other experts, the media. You just can't meet everyone's expectations, and you have to accept that.

What is the best part?

It is great being in an agency where everyone's passionate about the same thing that I'm passionate about. We're making a difference in people's lives on a grand scale, specifically targeting their health. Another great thing is having the opportunity to collaborate with people not just here at the CDC, but all over the country.

What advice do you have for someone who is interested in your career?

If you're not happy with what you're doing in medicine, and you're interested in public health, have the courage to make a change. It is not the typical path for an MD, and going against what's typical can be intimidating—but don't be afraid to try it. Keep an open mind, be flexible, be willing to move around and explore your interests.

PUBLIC HEALTH NURSE

Job Description

Although most nurses are trained to care for patients one-on-one, public health nurses do everything from providing direct care to leading community assessments and guiding policy change. They can be consultants, administrators, managers, and even leaders of health departments. A public health nurse involved in infectious disease control might run a sexually transmitted infection (STI) clinic, keep track of epidemiologic data on STIs in the community, and lead interventions in response to local trends. There are public health nurses who identify and track TB cases, and others who coordinate immunization clinics. When a disease outbreak occurs, public health nurses help investigate cases, speaking to patients and gathering information.

Public health nurses also work in many areas besides infectious disease prevention and control. Some make home visits and do case management for populations with certain health concerns. Some are involved in designing and carrying out health education programs, advocating for better health policies and laws, planning for emergencies and disasters, and other population-level health efforts.

Education and Certification

A public health nurse needs a current state nursing license. There are nurses doing public health work who have associates degrees, Bachelor of Science in Nursing (BSN) degrees, Master of Science in Nursing (MSN) degrees, and even PhDs. Leadership roles usually require at least a BSN. An MPH is very useful for a public health nursing career, and some nursing schools offer combined MSN/MPH programs. California and Minnesota have special requirements for public health nurses, although most states do not.

Core Competencies and Skills

- Passion for social justice
- Interest in community-level health
- Understanding of social issues within target populations
- Desire to work collaboratively across health disciplines
- Interest in health care policy
- Ability to make independent judgments
- Knowledge of both clinical and public health issues
- Knowledge of epidemiologic principles and techniques

Compensation

In 2008, the median salary for all nurses was about $62,000, with most earning between $43,000 and $92,000. Salaries for public health nurses depend on location, tasks, and experience. At one state health department, the salary range for a public health nurse at the supervisory level is about $55,000 to $84,000.

Workplaces

Many public health nurses work for city, county and state health departments, in a wide range of roles including infectious disease surveillance and control. There are opportunities at federal agencies, where public health nurses can contribute their knowledge to programs and policies on the national level. Public health nurses in the IHS provide direct service to patients as well as community assessment and intervention, and there are public health nurses serving as coordinators in the Women, Infant and Children (WIC) supplemental nutrition program. There are also jobs at nonprofit organizations, and there are public health nurses who are doctoral-level researchers and professors at universities.

Employment Outlook

Nurses make up a large proportion of the public health workforce, but according to a 2007 report from the Association of State and Territorial Health Officers (ASTHO), there is a severe shortage of public health nurses. The actual job description can vary; in some places, "public health nurses" are thought of more as workers in community clinics than as experts on population-level prevention and health promotion. However, there may be expanding opportunities for nurses who are specifically trained in public health.

For Further Information

- Association of State and Territorial Directors of Nursing (ASTDN) *www.astdn.org*
- American Public Health Association—Public Health Nursing Section *www.apha.org/membergroups/sections/aphasections/phn*
- Association of Community Health Nurse Educators (ACHNE) *www.achne.org*

PUBLIC HEALTH PROFILE: Public Health Nurse
Donna Westawski, MSN

Tuberculosis Nurse Consultant
Pennsylvania Department of Health, Wilkes-Barre, PA

Describe the sort of work you do.

I'm in charge of TB surveillance and management for a district within a state health department. Each state has communicable disease laws, telling what diseases need to be reported, and TB is one of those diseases. We need to find all of the active cases of TB that exist at any point in time, so that we can prevent transmission and make sure people are getting the right treatment. I'm involved in case finding, case management, surveillance, education and training, consulting, and the enforcement of regulations and communicable disease laws. I also maintain a registry of diagnosed cases, and I coordinate the schedule for directly observed therapy (DOT). DOT involves sending someone out to see certain patients each day, to make sure they take their medicine. If a patient refuses to be treated or to stay isolated until he is no longer contagious, we can use legal channels to have that person quarantined.

What is a typical day like at your job?

A large part of my day is working with the state's electronic reporting and surveillance system. Sometimes doctors call to report cases, but surveillance also means hunting and researching and looking for clues that there might be someone out there who has TB. The clue might be an abnormal chest x-ray, it might be a laboratory report. Automated reports from laboratories come in several times a day.

The same electronic reporting system is also a case management system. The CDC needs certain types of information about patients with TB. I enter data about risk factors, test results, treatment regimens and doses, and interim chest x-rays.

Another thing I do is handle telephone consultations. Some days I get no calls, and some days I get 20. A doctor might call about a patient whose medication is not agreeing with him. I often consult with nursing homes about what to do if a patient is confirmed as

Continued

having TB. We get a lot of calls from the general public, too. Other tasks include doing trainings for health care providers, testing people for TB, and helping with other health issues that come up in our community.

What education or training do you have? Is it typical for your job?

I have a BSN and a master's in community health nursing. The exact requirements for public health nurses differ from place to place.

What path did you take to get to the job you are in today?

I started with a 3-year diploma nursing program. I worked for a short time in clinical nursing. While I was doing that, I went on and earned my bachelor's degree. That's when I learned about public health nursing, because we had a rotation in community health. It was just a couple of years after finishing the baccalaureate program that I started working for the health department. I took several years off to raise a family, and during that time I earned a master's degree in community health nursing. I also did some teaching at 4-year nursing schools and worked part-time at a home health agency. After finishing the MSN, I completed a civil service application and put my name on a list for positions in public health nursing. Some time after that, when the health department was hiring, they called me in to interview.

Where might you go from here, if you wanted to advance your career?

There's not much advancement in my specific job. As a community health nurse, I could become a supervisor or administrator, running a larger program. If I considered anything else, I'd probably consider teaching again.

What is the worst or most challenging part of your job?

There are gray areas in TB diagnosis. Sometimes, my experience tells me that a particular patient does have TB and we need to take care

Continued

of him, but I can't hand the doctor a piece of paper that tells her what to do.

What is the best part?

I like having enough information and knowledge to be a consultant. I find it gratifying that when people call with questions and concerns, I can give them an answer. Often they'll say, 'I wish I'd called you a month ago!"

What advice do you have for someone who is interested in your career?

The APHA public health nursing section is a good resource. I would also say, get some clinical experience before you look for your first public health job. Much of the work you will do in public health is independent. You won't necessarily have a lot of staff or mentors. So if you can work in some different types of nursing, get some experience and build up your knowledge, it can really help.

PUBLIC HEALTH VETERINARIAN

Job Description

Public health veterinarians focus on the interaction between human and animal health. Their jobs can range from inspecting livestock to influencing national policy. Public health veterinarians help protect our food supply, contribute to disaster preparedness efforts, create and enforce regulations for animal shelters, consult with emergency room physicians, and more. Many are involved in infectious disease prevention and control. Some assist with the review and approval of drugs, such as antibiotics, that are used in animals. Others work to monitor and prevent the spread of diseases that can be transmitted from animals to humans (such as rabies, Lyme disease, *Escherichia coli*, and many others.) At the USDA, veterinarians' roles include making sure that meat and poultry plants are producing safe food, inspecting animals being brought into the country, investigating disease outbreaks, and seeking new ways to prevent disease in both animals and humans.

Some public health veterinarians work primarily in offices or labs, while others carry out on-site inspections at farms, factories, ports, and border areas. The job usually involves regular hours; however, a public health veterinarian may need to respond to emergencies on weekends, holidays, or other off-hours.

Education and Certification

A public health veterinarian must have a Doctor of Veterinary Medicine (DVM) degree and, in most cases, must have a current license to practice. Specific public health training or experience is not always required; however, jobs that involve disease surveillance, program design, policy, and other population-level efforts require a strong understanding of epidemiology and other aspects of public health. Some veterinary schools offer combined DVM/MPH programs, and there are opportunities for postgraduate training, including residency programs in veterinary public health. Public health veterinarians can seek certification from the American College of Veterinary Preventive Medicine (ACPVM).

Core Competencies and Skills

- Creative thinking
- Ability to see problems from multiple angles
- Passion for preventing, not just treating, disease
- Interest in working as part of a team
- Good communication skills
- At least a basic understanding of statistics and epidemiology
- Knowledge of veterinary medicine from both individual and population perspectives

Compensation

Salary surveys generally don't separate out public health veterinarians from those who provide direct patient care. The U.S. Bureau of Labor Statistics lists the median salary for all veterinarians as $79,000 in 2008, with most earning between $47,000 and $144,000. According to the American Veterinary Medical Association, in 2007 the median salary for veterinarians working for state or local government was $94,000 per year. In federal government, the median salary was $97,000 per year. For comparison, the median for vets in private practice was about $91,000 per year. Specific salaries vary by location, job responsibilities, qualifications, and seniority.

Workplaces

Veterinarians involved in public health activities are employed by local and state health departments and by federal agencies including the USDA, FDA, CDC, EPA, DHS, and the Department of Defense. There are also jobs in private industry that use public health skills and techniques.

Employment Outlook

Overall, it is expected that there will be more job openings for veterinarians than there are qualified people to fill them. Fewer jobs are available in public health than in clinical practice, but veterinarians who enter the field can expect continued support for disease control programs and food and animal safety efforts. Concerns about the need to maintain our food supply and minimize animal diseases in the United States and around the world may lead to additional opportunities.

For Further Information

- National Association of State Public Health Veterinarians (NASPHV)
  www.nasphv.org
- American College of Veterinary Preventive Medicine (ACVPM)
  www.acvpm.org
- American Association of Public Health Veterinarians (AAPHV)
  www.aaphv.org

PUBLIC HEALTH ADVISOR

Job Description

The title "public health advisor" originally belonged to a team of CDC field workers with basic public health training who went out into local communities to identify and treat patients with STIs. The program later expanded to include TB control and many other issues. Today, public health advisors often come to the job through an extensive training fellowship. They are closely involved in program design and implementation, providing efficient response to public health needs. As public health advisors rise through the ranks, they gain more responsibility and may eventually manage large programs. Some public health advisors are stationed at federal agency headquarters; others are assigned to locations around the country or overseas, where they assist with local public health efforts.

Public health advisors are also found at other agencies and in other areas of public health. There are public health advisors working in disaster preparedness, nutrition, mental health, and many other areas of disease prevention and health promotion.

Education and Certification

A CDC public health advisor needs at least a bachelor's degree. One way to become eligible for a public health advisor job is to complete the CDC's Public Health Apprentice Program (PHAP) or Public Health Prevention Service (PHPS). PHAP is a 2-year fellowship in which recent college graduates are assigned to train at state and local health agencies. PHPS is a 3-year fellowship for master's level public health professionals. Higher-level jobs require appropriate experience.

Core Competencies and Skills

- Adaptability
- Initiative
- Good communication skills
- Knack for evaluating situations and determining what is needed
- Ability to apply research findings to practice
- Ability to make decisions independently, but also to collaborate with a team
- Strong understanding of the elements of public health practice, including the use of epidemiologic data, disease surveillance and control, and program design, implementation, and evaluation

Compensation

Public health advisors at the CDC start in the $50,000s to $60,000s, with adjustments for location. Experienced advisors with significant responsibility can reach $100,000, and there are senior-level positions with higher salaries.

Workplaces

Public health advisors have an important role at the CDC. There are also public health advisors at other federal agencies, including other departments within HHS and USAID. Some state and local agencies have similar job titles.

Employment Outlook

Public health advisors are well prepared for a wide range of public health activities. There are many opportunities for advancement, and the skills gained through this job tend to be in demand at state and local agencies and nonprofit organizations, as well.

For Further Information

■ Watsonian Society
www.cdc.gov/watsonian/default.htm

VACCINE RESEARCHER

Job Description

Vaccine researchers look at everything from how the immune system works to how to prevent specific diseases, like HIV/AIDS and malaria. Other issues include predicting who is likely to respond to a vaccine and figuring out how long the protection from a vaccine will last. There are researchers working to improve upon existing vaccines, too—to deliver better protection or make immunity last longer.

Some vaccine researchers examine immune responses on the cellular or molecular level. Some test potential new vaccines in human populations. Some study the safety of vaccines. In general, vaccine researchers must have a strong understanding of the immune system, of the processes involved in infection, and of how vaccines are thought to work. In addition, researchers may write journal articles, present results at conferences, help write medical textbooks, and even give advice to policy makers.

Education and Certification

A researcher who wants to run a laboratory or be primarily responsible for designing and carrying out studies related to vaccines needs a doctoral degree, usually a PhD, followed by additional postdoctoral training. Typical fields for the PhD include molecular biology, immunology, microbiology, or biochemistry, although the name of the degree is less important than the actual topics studied. Some vaccine researchers are MDs who have additional training and experience in research.

Core Competencies and Skills

- Understanding of the scientific method
- Good attention to detail and an appreciation for precision
- Strong sense of ethics, especially when human or animal subjects are involved
- Ability to work as part of a team
- Patience and the ability to accept that studies may not give hoped-for results
- Knowledge specific to infectious diseases and the immune system
- Practical skills for the design and implementation of clinical or laboratory studies.

Compensation

According to national statistics, the median salary for a medical scientist, a job category that includes people involved in developing vaccines, is about $73,000. However, many researchers earn substantially more. A typical starting salary for the head of a laboratory at a federal agency is around $100,000, and people in senior positions can reach $200,000 per year or more. Research professors can expect similar compensation levels, although it varies from one university to another. PhDs in postdoctoral positions start at lower salaries, with a jump to higher salaries in their first jobs after this level.

Workplaces

Vaccine research is carried out at multiple places including NIH and university departments. The U.S. Army Research Institute on Infectious

Diseases also develops vaccines, primarily to protect service members from potential biological warfare agents and dangerous endemic diseases.

Employment Outlook

The need for medical scientists with doctoral-level degrees is expected to increase over the next several years, and people with both an MD and PhD should be particularly in demand. However, competition for individual jobs is typical in research fields. In addition, a job will often require a very specific background, and it may be a challenge to find a position that matches one's training and interests. The availability of federal funding will also influence the number of jobs available in both government and academic settings.

For Further Information

- Vaccine Research Center at the National Institute of Allergy and Infectious Disease
  www3.niaid.nih.gov/about/organization/vrc
- National Foundation for Infectious Diseases (NFID)
  www.nfid.org
- The International Vaccine Institute (IVI)
  www.ivi.org

PUBLIC HEALTH PROFILE: Vaccine Researcher
Mario Roederer, PhD

Senior Investigator, ImmunoTechnology Section
Vaccine Research Center, National Institute of Allergy and Infectious Diseases, National Institutes of Health, Bethesda, MD

Describe the sort of work you do.

I'm in charge of a research laboratory at the Vaccine Research Center. In my laboratory, we're exploring how immune responses develop. That's important for understanding and treating natural infections, and it is also important for developing vaccines. Every time you test a vaccine, it takes thousands of people, millions of dollars, and several

Continued

years, so you want to start with a vaccine that is likely to have a good protective response. But at this point, we don't really know which immune system responses are the most likely to be protective. We are trying to determine that, so we can develop vaccines more quickly.

What is a typical day like at your job?

I supervise about a dozen people. My day typically involves providing them with advice on how to design experiments and interpret data, and helping them write up the results for publication. I also participate in outside advisory activities, and sometimes we collaborate with people who are developing similar research programs. There is administrative work, as well. And I go to a number of conferences. At my level, I don't do direct laboratory work. Some people make the choice to stay in the lab. I'd rather focus on providing the best advice and input.

What education or training do you have? Is it typical for your job?

Everyone's a little different. My PhD is in cell biology, and my background is more hard science and technical than most people in my position. I'm an adept computer programmer, I know physics and chemistry ... so we do a lot of technology development in my lab, not just application.

You need a PhD or MD to do my job, and you need additional experience. It takes a lot of years to really learn how to run a laboratory and how to organize it. You also have to think globally—how the different experiments tie together.

What path did you take to get to the job you are in today?

As is often the case in the research world, finding my current job at the NIH was a matter of good timing. The Vaccine Research Center was just being created. I was told by a colleague that they were looking for someone with a background like mine. Usually, for this type of job, there is just one opening and a lot of people apply for it.

Continued

I applied, not expecting to get the job—and I did get it. It was an outstanding opportunity, a perfect fit for the research I was envisioning.

Where might you go from here, if you wanted to advance your career?

I'm right where I want to be right now, so I would characterize a change not as a step up, but as a step in a different direction. Some people might want to run a department or run an institute. At that point, though, you're not really doing science anymore. It is much more administrative. You could do science policy, you could work for a foundation and do research grants, you could work for a biotech company. There's not one single career ladder.

What is the worst or most challenging part of your job?

My calendar is much more full than it used to be, with conference calls and meetings. I understand the necessity of those, and I even enjoy them—but I don't have the freedom I used to. My job also calls for a lot of traveling. I enjoy the travel, but it gets hard, especially when you have a family. It's hard being away from the lab, too.

What is the best part?

My joy is enabling science, helping research happen. And I love giving presentations. It's my chance to tell people about the cool things that we do!

What advice do you have for someone who is interested in your career?

You have to experience it. When you're in school, spend some time in the laboratory and discover what it is like to spend 60 or 70 hours a week there. Get into it thinking that you will give it a shot—but it is not for everyone. There are a lot more postdoctoral jobs than there are faculty, and it's partly because people realize this work is not for them. You have to have a love for it!

DISEASE ECOLOGIST

Job description

Disease ecologists study patterns of diseases in populations, with an emphasis on understanding the principles that underlie disease patterns. They look at interactions of populations with each other and with the environment, and ask how those interactions influence the emergence of new diseases, the spread of familiar ones, and the appearance of outbreaks and epidemics. Some disease ecologists study the evolution of drug resistance and virulence among infectious agents, and the development of resistance to infection among potential hosts (such as humans).

Not all disease ecologists do work that is likely to inform public health directly. However, there are some ecologists studying how climate change is likely to impact infectious disease in human populations, how environmental changes may contribute to the emergence of new diseases, and how biodiversity can influence the risk of diseases in humans. Some are directly involved in investigating outbreaks and creating policies to prevent disease. Some work largely with computer models or in laboratories, while others do field research.

Education and Certification

Disease ecologists generally have PhDs or other doctoral degrees. There are now some university departments specializing in disease ecology, but infectious disease ecology, especially, is still an emerging field. Many established disease ecologists earned their PhDs in fields such as microbiology, ecology, entomology, or zoology, and some are veterinarians. There are a few roles in applied disease ecology for people with BS or MS degrees.

Core Competencies and Skills

- Curiosity
- Persistence
- Ability to collaborate with people who have different types of expertise
- Ability to communicate complex ideas on paper and in person
- Interest not only in clinical manifestations of disease, causes, or risk factors, but also in what causes patterns of disease to occur
- Appreciation of the interactions among epidemiology, ecology, genetics, and medicine

- Good math and statistical skills and an understanding of how research is designed and carried out
- Willingness to work both in the laboratory and in the field

Compensation

Because "disease ecologist" can refer to people from many different disciplines, there are no national salary statistics. In 2008, the median salary for professors in the biological sciences was about $71,000 and for environmental sciences, $65,000. Low-end salaries were in the $30 to $40,000 range and high-end salaries in the low to mid-$100,000s. Variations in salaries make it hard to compare academic and non-academic jobs, but microbiologists who were not also educators had a median salary of about $65,000, with most earning $38,000 to $111,000; salaries for zoologists and wildlife biologists tended to be a little lower. (These numbers include jobs with various responsibilities and areas of focus, not just disease ecologists.)

Workplaces

Disease ecologists focusing on public health issues work at universities, including schools of public health, at nonprofit organizations that support research, and at government agencies including USGS, CDC, USDA, and some state health departments. There are also opportunities at organizations that do work in the developing world.

Employment Outlook

Competition for jobs varies. Recent PhD graduates may find it challenging to locate a job that matches their specific research interests, but attending scientific meetings and networking with others in the field is often a good way to find opportunities.

For Further Information

- The Ecological Society of America (ESA)
  www.esa.org
- Society for Vector Ecology (SOVE)
  www.sove.org

■ American Society for Tropical Medicine and Hygiene (ASTMH)
  www.astmh.org

INFECTION PREVENTIONIST

Job Description

Infection preventionists are experts on practical methods of preventing and controlling the spread of infectious diseases, typically within a specific population—the patients, staff, and visitors at a hospital or other health care setting. Their work also helps reduce the risk of contagious diseases being carried out into the community. Infection control practices include surveillance, investigation of cases and outbreaks, training of staff members, the development and enforcement of infection control policies, and evaluation of the effectiveness of infection control efforts. If an outbreak occurs, infection preventionists track down the source and control the problem. They must be alert to any unusual illness that could signal an outbreak, a new type of infection, or even the first casualty of a bioterrorism attack. They spend some time collecting and analyzing data, but they also observe staff members' practices, participate in patient rounds, attend meetings, and design and lead interventions to improve infection control.

Some infection preventionists are involved in protecting the health of wider communities. They may provide guidance on controlling epidemics, protecting against emerging diseases, or planning in case of a bioterrorism attack. Many infection preventionists in health care settings have additional responsibilities, such as employee health. (To learn more about jobs in patient safety, see chapter 18.)

Education and Certification

Requirements depend on the specific job setting. Many infection preventionists are RNs. Some have MPH degrees or other relevant training. Although special certification is not necessarily required, job candidates may be viewed more favorably if they have a CIC certification (Certified in Infection Control), which is obtained by passing a test administered by the Certification Board of Infection Control and Epidemiology. There are also infectious disease physicians and PhDs whose work focuses on infection control.

Core Competencies and Skills

- Curiosity and persistence
- Good problem solving skills and the ability to think creatively
- Ability to make timely decisions, using good judgment
- Understanding of epidemiology and data analysis techniques
- Strong enough science background to understand how infections are transmitted and what protective practices are appropriate in a given situation
- Knowledge of infection control guidelines and regulations
- Good understanding of human behavior, to understand how and why people put themselves at risk

Compensation

Salaries vary depending on specific qualifications, responsibilities, and location. According to a 2006 survey of members of the Association for Professionals in Infection Control and Epidemiology (APIC), the majority of whom were nurses, about half were earning salaries in the range of $50,000 to $75,000. Twenty-one percent were in the lower range of $30,000 to $50,000, and 20% made $75,000 a year or more. Most survey respondents worked directly in health care settings; about 5% had jobs specifically in public health. Physicians who are involved in infection control often have other responsibilities as well, so their salaries are more in keeping with others in their specialty.

Workplaces

Infection preventionists can be found at hospitals and outpatient centers, as well as hospices, home-care organizations, and other settings where health services are provided. Health departments, federal agencies, nonprofit organizations, and university centers also employ these experts to enhance infection control practices on a wider scale. Some infection preventionists work with the military, and some are even involved in global health, such as working to prevent outbreaks in developing countries.

Employment Outlook

With a growing emphasis on patient safety, hospitals are paying increasing attention to infection control and job opportunities are very good. In addition, many current infection preventionists are nearing retirement age. Current concerns about bioterrorism and emerging diseases also provide opportunities for these specialists.

For Further Information

■ Association for Professionals in Infection Control and Epidemiology (APIC)
www.apic.org

5 Chronic Disease and Cancer

Chronic disease is an increasingly important concern in the world of public health. The number of Americans with type 2 diabetes has soared in recent years. Heart disease is the leading cause of death in the United States. Asthma affects more than 16 million adults and 7 million children. About one-fifth of children and one-quarter of adults have untreated dental cavities. Cancer, which many health professionals also classify as a chronic disease, is the second leading cause of death in the United States.

There are ways to reduce the risk and lessen the impact of many chronic diseases, but often we don't take advantage of them. Regular exercise and a healthful diet have numerous benefits, but a lot of us don't follow the recommended guidelines. And many people with chronic diseases don't get the care they need.

Public health asks what we can change in our neighborhoods, our communities, and our health care system to get better control of chronic diseases. Some experts focus on measuring disease incidence and prevalence and tracking patterns in different communities. Others look at what can be done. Do people need education about healthy choices? Is there something we can alter in the environment, like prohibiting smoking in restaurants or posting calorie information on menus? Do we need to train doctors to provide better care? Is there a way to ensure that people who need treatment are getting it?

In this chapter, you'll learn about some careers involving chronic disease prevention and intervention. To learn about others, see the descriptions for epidemiologist, medical officer, public health nurse, environmental health nurse, nutritionist, corporate medical director, and community activist, and the chapters on Maternal and Child Health, Vulnerable and At-Risk Populations, and Health Research. The CDC has a Web site devoted to chronic disease prevention and health promotion at www.cdc.gov/chronicdisease.

HEALTH EDUCATOR

Job Description

Health educators convey health information to the public in ways that people will understand—and, ideally, find interesting and useful, too. They begin by figuring out what people in a given community do and do not know about a particular health topic. In chronic disease prevention, this might be preventing diabetes, controlling asthma, or detecting colon cancer. (Health educators may also teach about many other topics besides chronic disease.) They determine how most people in that community like to learn and what will catch their attention. For example, pamphlets might be good for college students who like to read, but not very useful in an inner-city community where literacy is low. Next, they put together programs—classes, videos, even cell phone texts—that convey the needed information. When possible, they follow up by evaluating the success of the program, to see what people learned and if their behavior or health changed as a result.

Health educators are involved in all levels of health promotion, from designing local programs to serving as advisors for national health campaigns. In addition to teaching members of the general public, in some places they work on systems-level programs, such as teaching convenience store owners how they can stock healthier foods.

Education and Certification

A bachelor's degree is the minimum qualification to work as a health educator; degrees in health education are available, but another degree plus related experience or training will often suffice. A master's degree, such as an MPH with specialization in public or community health education, broadens the job possibilities and contributes to the chances for advancement. Certification as a Certified Health Education Specialist, which requires an exam administered by the National Commission for Health Education Credentialing (NCHEC), is preferred for many public health jobs and occasionally is required.

Core Competencies and Skills

- Knack for explaining complex information in a straightforward, easily understandable way
- At least basic knowledge of health and medicine, and the ability to understand medical information
- Excellent spoken and written communication skills
- Appreciation of cultural diversity
- Understanding of human psychology and behavior
- Ability to create a curriculum covering necessary information
- Understanding of research processes and survey design
- Ability to write for people with low reading literacy and low health literacy

Compensation

In 2008, the average salary for a health educator was $49,000. Most earned between $26,000 and $78,000.

Workplaces

Health educators who create and implement public health programs are found in government agencies, nonprofit organizations, college and universities, and sometimes hospitals and medical centers. (In medical settings, they are more likely to provide one-on-one teaching.)

Employment Outlook

Over the next few years, the number of jobs for health educators and the number of qualified job seekers are expected to be in balance. Rising interest in the prevention of disease as a way to control health care costs may lead to more opportunities.

For Further Information

- Society for Public Health Education (SOPHE)
  www.sophe.org
- American Public Health Association—Public Health Education and
  Health Promotion section
  www.apha.org/membergroups/sections/aphasections/phehp
- American Association for Health Education (AAHE)
  www.aahperd.org/AAHE

HEALTH PROMOTION PROGRAM COORDINATOR

Job Description

Health promotion programs can be local, state-level, or nationwide efforts
to get people to adopt healthier behaviors. Examples include the national
"5 A Day" campaign to remind people to eat their fruits and veggies; a small-
town program that helps migrant workers get access to health care; smoking cessation hotlines; condom distribution programs; and "fit city" exercise
campaigns. There are programs that encourage corner grocery stores to
carry healthier foods and doctors to talk to their patients about smoking.

Each of these programs has a coordinator or manager (or sometimes
more than one) to oversee everything from the planning process, to the
daily activities, to the analysis of data that's collected. Responsibilities can
include developing educational materials, partnering with other organizations, raising funds, hiring and firing employees, reaching out to the media,
and making sure that the program is running smoothly. In small programs,
the coordinator may do all these things directly; in larger programs, a director will delegate tasks to employees.

This is primarily an office job, with the usual business hours. Program
coordinators may also need to attend evening meetings, be present at
weekend events or conferences, and visit community sites. Late hours
may sometimes be needed to meet a grant deadline, prepare a report, or
respond to media interest.

Education and Certification

A program coordinator usually has at least a bachelor's degree. A master's degree in public health or a related field is often required. There
is no special certification required for this job, but for larger programs,
especially, relevant experience is expected.

Core Competencies and Skills

- Good public speaking and presentation skills
- Strong management skills
- Excellent social skills for interacting with program participants and leaders of other programs and organizations
- Strong writing skills
- Understanding of the population that the program serves
- Knowledge of how to apply research results to real-world programs

Compensation

Compensation depends on experience, on the size of the program, and on the budget of the agency or organization. Many jobs, particularly with small organizations or small programs, have salaries in the $40,000 to $50,000 range. Program coordinators can eventually become directors at programs with statewide or national reach, with higher salaries to match the level of responsibility.

Workplaces

Health promotion program coordinators usually work for academic institutions, government agencies, and nonprofits, or for consulting firms that serve these types of organizations.

Employment Outlook

Jobs are most likely to be available in cities and counties with larger and more active health departments, with corporations that are based nearby and have taken an interest in a particular situation, or with local foundations that have a special interest in promoting public health. Health promotion programs are often grant-funded and may continue for only a limited number of years, but new programs are often being launched, as well.

For Further Information

- American Public Health Association—Public Health Education and Health Promotion section
  www.apha.org/membergroups/sections/aphasections/phehp

PUBLIC HEALTH PROFILE: Health Promotion Program Coordinator
John Wedeles, MPH
Program Coordinator
Manhattan Tobacco Cessation Program, New York, NY

Describe the sort of work do you do.

I am the Program Coordinator for the Manhattan Tobacco Cessation Program (MTCP), one of 19 cessation centers throughout New York State. MTCP is funded by the New York State Department of Health. My job is to give health care providers (doctors, nurses, nurse practitioners, and medical assistants) the knowledge and resources to help their patients successfully quit smoking. MTCP promotes the "5 As" model, which recommends that providers ask about tobacco use, advise smokers to quit, assess their readiness to quit, assist them in their attempt to quit by referring them to cessation services or prescribing pharmacotherapy, and arrange a follow-up visit. We also help clinics develop their paper charts or electronic medical records so that tobacco treatment becomes a standard practice. And we supply them with educational resources for both providers and patients.

What is a typical day like at your job?

During a typical day, I work on collecting or analyzing data from patient charts to determine whether a partner site is adhering to the 5 As model. I'll summarize the data and point out achievements, areas where improvements can be made, and so on. I might advise a hospital or clinic about larger policy issues, such as smoke-free grounds. I also might give a training to clinic staff on practicing the 5 As. I represent my group at a community health fairs, too, distributing educational materials and answering questions.

What education or training do you have? Is it typical for your job?

I have a master's degree in public health. Most of my colleagues have master's degrees in public health or public administration. Several have clinical backgrounds, including a few who are registered nurses.

Continued

Also I'm a trained tobacco treatment specialist. While I don't provide direct patient care, the training gave me an excellent background in tobacco treatment that I use in my staff trainings for partner sites.

What path did you take to get to the job you are in today?

After two jobs in marketing and public affairs, I switched careers and started working as a public affairs assistant for a hospital trade association. I also volunteered at a hospital in order to strengthen my background in health care, with the intention of going to graduate school in public administration or public health. Once I got to graduate school, I volunteered for MTCP. The program coordinator position opened up shortly after I graduated, and at that point they already knew me and liked my work.

Where might you go from here, if you wanted to advance your career?

From here, I could continue in program management in more of an administrative role. Because I do a fair amount of data collection and analysis, I could also seek a position at a research organization. A job at a consulting firm might be a good fit as well.

What is the worst or most challenging part of your job?

Many of the health care providers I work with are often pressed for time. As a result, treating tobacco use is sometimes not a high priority in comparison to other health conditions. In addition, sometimes it is easy to get caught up in the daily tasks without having an eye for long-term strategy and goals. It is essential to always be thinking 6 months down the road and looking at how your daily work will meet your annual deliverables.

What is the best part?

I've been able to impart real change to the partner sites I work with. In certain instances, following a staff training, we have observed improvements in the doctors' adherence to the 5 As. We've also requested changes to the electronic medical record template at the Pediatric clinics, which led to improvements in adherence. Another

Continued

great part about my job is the variety of activities—from research and data collection to training to policy development.

What advice would you give to someone who wanted to do this type of work?

For this particular job, I would tell that person to get trained as a tobacco treatment specialist, so you have those skills to pass on to health care providers. It also helps to have experience in a clinical setting to understand the flow of patient care. A master's degree in public health or public administration will be very helpful as well. Public health is all about collaboration, so I would be open to partnering with other organizations, administrative departments—anything that will help open doors throughout your work.

MEDICAL EPIDEMIOLOGIST/CHRONIC DISEASE

Job Description

Medical epidemiologists are public health physicians who bring a strong knowledge of clinical medicine to their epidemiology work. (See the description of epidemiologist to learn more.) Their medical training gives them special understanding of the clinical manifestations of diseases, the underlying pathophysiology, the ways medications work, and the nuances that can make the study of certain diseases especially complex. Medical epidemiologists can do surveillance and monitoring, outbreak investigation, and research, not just in chronic disease (such as asthma, cardiovascular disease, diabetes, and cancer), but in all areas of public health. Some use their skills to help design and evaluate disease prevention programs. Often, medical epidemiologists serve as consultants to nonphysician epidemiologists and other public health experts. They also have the knowledge to talk peer-to-peer with other physicians about medical information. Some medical epidemiologists are specialists, focusing on one area of health, others are generalists.

Education and Certification

In most cases, a medical epidemiologist must have an MD or DO degree. Many jobs also require completion of a residency program and a license to practice, and some require a specific medical specialty. It is possible to do epidemiologic work without specialized training, but employers usually prefer or require an MPH degree, completion of the EIS program, or other relevant education.

Core Competencies and Skills

- Curiosity about patterns of disease
- Logical and analytical thinking
- Creativity
- Ability to explain medical knowledge to nonphysicians
- Strong knowledge of epidemiologic principles
- Knowledge of how to use statistics programs and databases
- Good background in clinical medicine, an interest in learning more, and the ability to search and understand the medical literature

Compensation

Salaries vary by level, experience, and location. In the federal government, physicians doing public health work can earn from around $72,000 to $150,000 or more; salaries increase with experience and responsibility. Overall, salaries in the range of $95,000 to $150,000 are common.

Workplaces

Medical epidemiologists work for local and state health departments and for federal agencies including the CDC, the NIH, and the Department of Defense. Some are university faculty. There are also opportunities at nonprofit organizations and in consulting firms.

Employment Outlook

There is expanding interest in epidemiologic approaches to chronic disease, maternal and child health, substance abuse, disaster preparedness, and other topics beyond the more traditional focus on infectious disease. This may lead to new opportunities for medical epidemiologists. In general, the number of jobs for epidemiologists is expected to increase over the next few years.

For Further Information

- See the listings under the entries for epidemiologist and medical officer.

PUBLIC HEALTH PROFILE: Medical Epidemiologist
Sarah Schillie
Medical Epidemiologist
U.S. Public Health Service Commissioned Corps
Centers for Disease Control and Prevention, Springfield, IL

Describe the sort of work you do.

I'm a medical doctor with special training in public health and epidemiology. I'm an officer in the U.S. Public Health Service Commissioned Corps and am employed by the CDC. Currently I'm a chronic disease field epidemiology assignee to the Illinois Department of Public Health, so I am employed by the federal government but work at the state level.

My job is multifaceted, but most of my work revolves around asthma, tobacco, and obesity. I design evaluations for chronic disease programs and interventions, analyze and interpret surveillance data, and collaborate with other agencies to develop public health interventions. Part of my assignment is to help build epidemiologic capacity within the state, which includes teaching others about epidemiologic principles and methods.

What is a typical day like at your job?

A typical day includes working with data, writing, providing technical assistance, and attending meetings. The data analyses range from simple, descriptive statistics to more complex analysis. The writing includes reports, abstracts, and press releases. I provide guidance to co-workers and stakeholders on things such as survey design, data analysis, and data interpretation. My participation in meetings often involves providing subject matter expertise or presentations.

Project managers often ask me to display data using maps. For example, I recently created state maps depicting obesity rates by county over time. Additionally, I spend quite a bit of time creating web-based surveys. I'm currently working on an electronic survey as part of an evaluation for various asthma interventions that are conducted by grantees.

Continued

What education or training do you have? Is it typical for your job?

I have an MD and an MPH, and recently received an MBA. After medical school I completed residencies in pediatrics and preventive medicine, as well as the 2-year EIS program at the CDC. The medical training provided me with a broad-based background, and also allows for additional flexibility regarding my assignments. For example, in the event of a public health emergency I could respond in several different capacities. The preventive medicine, public health, and epidemiology training provided me with important skillsets necessary to perform my duties. The MBA is somewhat unique for public health work, but that education has impacted the way I think about allocating resources and implementing processes to improve efficiency.

What path did you take to get to the job you are in today?

After my residency training, I worked as the Director of Performance Improvement at a county health department for 4 years. I think that experience has helped to keep me grounded and remember the true meaning of public health. I left that job to enter the EIS program, and this is my first assignment after completing EIS.

Where might you go from here, if you wanted to advance your career?

One of the advantages of being part of the U.S. Public Health Service Commissioned Corps is mobility, including mobility in terms of federal agency, subject area, and geography. As far as advancing one's career, my philosophy has always been that it's important to get as many different experiences as possible, and also a wide variety of experiences.

What is the worst or most challenging part of your job?

There is a lot of paperwork. Although it is not challenging from an intellectual standpoint, it can be frustrating and time-consuming.

What is the best part?

The work impacts the health of populations, which I believe is a very noble cause. There is also much variety with public health work, and

Continued

for the most part it is rewarding, intellectually stimulating, and fascinating. Also, the field of public health tends to attract genuinely good people, so having wonderful co-workers has been another advantage.

What advice do you have for someone who is interested in your career?

The importance of a diversity of public health-related experiences early on cannot be over-emphasized, and those experiences could be gained from academia, government, or a nonprofit organization. My advice would be to learn as many skills as possible, including statistical software and survey design. The ability to communicate in another language, such as Spanish, would always be helpful. And finally, become adept at public speaking.

PUBLIC HEALTH DENTIST

Job Description

Public health dentists often combine direct patient care with work focusing on population-level health. Some provide services to patients in underserved areas or those who could not afford dental care otherwise. They are also administrators, advisors, and consultants, helping to create and oversee programs that provide care or promote dental health. There are public health dentists involved in programs such as community water fluoridation, school-based dental screenings, oral cancer screenings, and educational efforts to promote good oral hygiene. Some advise politicians on new programs that should be funded and enacted. Some participate in forensic investigations, using their skills to help identify victims of crimes or disasters.

Education and Certification

Public health dentists need a Doctor of Dental Medicine (DMD) or Doctor of Dental Surgery (DDS) degree and a license to practice in the state where they work. Extra training may not be needed, but experience or training in the world of public health is often expected. Many public health dentists hold MPH degrees. Dentists can pursue residency training specifically in dental public health, which includes earning an MPH, and obtain specialty board certification from the American Board of Dental Public Health.

Core Competencies and Skills

- Strong leadership, management, and communication skills
- Ability to work with a team that may include other health professionals, community leaders, politicians, researchers, and others
- Ability to design, manage, and evaluate community programs
- Interest in research and the knowledge of how to design and carry out studies
- Understanding of epidemiologic principles and at least basic statistics
- Up-to-date knowledge of dental health, oral hygiene practices, and preventive dentistry

Compensation

A typical salary for a public health dentist is similar to what a general dentist would earn. The median salary for dentists in general practice is $143,000, with most earning at least $72,000 per year. For public health dentists who work at universities, salaries range from about $50,000 per year to about $200,000 for the very highest level jobs. Public health dentists usually have positions that include benefits such as health insurance and retirement plans, unlike dentists in private practice.

Workplaces

Many health departments employ public health dentists to work in community clinics and/or to develop policy and oversee oral health programs. A small number work at the CDC. Some are professors at dental schools.

Employment Outlook

The number of board-certified public health dentists is small, and less than 1% of U.S. dentists work in public health. At present, there appear to be more public health dentistry jobs than there are qualified public health dentists.

For Further Information

■ American Association of Public Health Dentistry (AAPHD)
www.aaphd.org
■ Association of State and Territorial Dental Directors (ASTDD)
www.astdd.org
■ American Public Health Association—Oral Health Section
www.apha.org/membergroups/sections/aphasections/oral

PUBLIC HEALTH PROFILE: Public Health Dentist
James Lalumandier, DDS, MPH
Professor and Chair of Community Dentistry
Case Western Reserve University School of Dental Medicine,
Cleveland, OH

Describe the sort of work you do.

As a public health dentist in an academic position, there are three
elements to what I do: research, teaching, and service. What I like
to do the most revolves around teaching and service. When I started
at my current job, there was a small sealant program serving kids in
the public schools. (Dental sealant is a material that helps prevent
cavities.) Our program sends dental students into schools in low-
income neighborhoods to do exams, administer sealant, and teach
children about oral hygiene. I've worked to expand the program,
and now each year over 20,000 school children are educated, over
6,000 treated and approximately 3,000 referred for additional
treatment.

What is a typical day like at your job?

When I was setting up the program, on a typical day I would be bringing equipment out to schools, meeting with principals and teachers,
instructing dental students and dental hygiene students, and talking
to the children. Then I'd oversee the dental students doing the exams
and applying the sealant. To get the program into the dental school

Continued

curriculum, I had to write out exactly what was planned, what the students would do, what they would learn, and why it was important to their education. I also had to obtain funding, which meant looking for opportunities, networking, and writing proposals for grants. Now, I have two full-time health educators to teach the children, two part-time dentists and eight additional personnel; therefore, my role in the program is primarily administrative.

What education or training do you have? Is it typical for your job?

I have a DDS and an MPH degree, and I'm board-certified in dental public health. There are a lot of very good public health dentists who don't have an MPH, but I would recommend it. Most schools of public heath don't have a dental track, but you can choose a dental school that has a public health track.

What path did you take to get to the job you are in today?

After dental school, I did a general practice residency through a military program. I went back into the military to get public health training, including an MPH. After I retired from the military, I worked for 2 years at a health department. I had been thinking that community dentistry was something I would love to do, so when I heard about an opening for Chair of Community Health Dentistry at the dental school, I applied for the job. Doing general dentistry would probably not have been enough to qualify for the position, but I already had an MPH with a scholarly record of peer reviewed publications. I was also board certified in my specialty, and there are only about 150 boarded public health dentists in the United States.

When I first took this job, colleagues said that taking on the sealant program was not a good idea. In academia, publications are very important, and running a program could limit the number of research papers I could publish. But this is what I wanted to do, and it has turned out very well.

Continued

Where might you go from here, if you wanted to advance your career?

If I were going to take a "next step," I'd want to be a dean. I'm not much into titles, but as a dean I could focus a dental school on access to care issues. Access to care is a real problem in dentistry. I'd like to devote a larger part of education to showing students how rewarding it is to work in very rural or urban areas, and to help those who need help the most.

What is the worst or most challenging part of your job?

My least favorite part of the job is the administrative stuff. I'd much rather be treating patients and making somebody's life a little better.

What is the best part?

The most fun is interacting with both the children and the students. It is helping the students to be better dentists, and hopefully inspiring some of them to look beyond private practice in suburbia. And it is educating the children to take care of their teeth and to feel comfortable with getting dental care.

What advice do you have for someone who is interested in your career?

Learn about what public health is. It is not right for everybody. Research it, find out what public health dentists do, and then if you're still interested, give it a shot!

TOBACCO QUITLINE ADVISOR

Job Description

At a tobacco "quitline," counselors take calls from members of the public who want to quit smoking. They help each caller make a plan for quitting and then follow up to see how they are doing. They use special interviewing techniques to increase motivation and guide callers through the quitting process. At some quitlines, the counselors can help callers obtain free nicotine patches or gum. Counselors keep records of calls and often are required to use a computerized charting system, which allows data to be collected for quality assurance and research. Some quitlines offer interactive, web-based services as well. Quitlines tend to be open from early morning to late at night, so counselors usually work either set hours or in shifts. There may be an option to work part-time or even from home.

Education and Certification

Quitline services generally look for people with at least a bachelor's degree. Some ask for training in social work, psychology, or another field that incorporates counseling, and some prefer counselors with master's degrees. There is usually on-the-job training in specific methods and techniques to be used.

Core Competencies and Skills

- Emotional stability
- Strong listening skills
- Patience and empathy to work with callers who may have multiple mental, emotional, or physical challenges
- Ability to help guide people toward finding their own solutions to problems
- Fluency in a language other English (not required but can be extremely helpful)
- Ability to follow a protocol and to use the counseling style directed by the helpline organization

Compensation

Quitline counselors are not highly paid, but it can be a fulfilling job. A starting salary of around $30,000 per year is not uncommon, with supervisors earning in the $40,000 to $50,000 range.

Workplaces

Quitline counselors work for nonprofit organizations, health departments, and universities. There are also for-profit organizations that run quitline services, both for health departments and for corporations.

Employment Outlook

Most states have at least one tobacco quitline, and there seems to be ongoing support for such services. Working as a quitline counselor can be a good entry-level opportunity for someone interested in health behavior or in direct-service programs. There are also helplines to assist with substance abuse, problem gambling, domestic violence, and other health issues (requirements for employment vary).

For Further Information

■ North American Quitline Consortium (NAQC)
  www.naquitline.org
■ *Smokefree.gov*

PUBLIC HEALTH PROFILE: Tobacco Quitline Advisor
Shelley Anderson
Counselor
California Smokers' Helpline, San Diego, CA

Describe the sort of work you do.

The purpose of my job is to give people the tools they need to be able to stop smoking and to provide extra support during the first couple of weeks while they are trying to quit. The California Smokers' Helpline aims to reach as many people as possible, so our protocol is fine-tuned to cover the most important key topics in a call lasting 20 to 30 minutes. We focus on motivation, planning, use of quit aids, and setting a quit date. We discuss any ambivalence the person might feel, help identify smoking triggers, and help callers come up with strategies to avoid or overcome those triggers. We talk about which quit aids might work best for a particular client and in many instances we can help them get their insurance to cover them. We encourage callers to at least *try* to quit.

What is a typical day like at your job?

I usually start taking calls right away. When people call for the first time, they can choose to get materials only, or choose materials and counseling.

Continued

Our goal is to try and move them right into a counseling call. We ask a series of questions to help determine how to best help them. We also collect demographic information which helps us know whom we are reaching throughout the state. If they want counseling but are not able to do it right on the spot, I set up an appointment and we call them back.

On slower days, I focus more on outgoing calls to clients we have not yet counseled, or clients we want to follow up with. Often, if someone has relapsed, we'll set a new quit date and start the process again. Though I try to cover the main points in our protocol, I can adjust the conversations to each individual caller.

What education or training do you have? Is it typical for your job?

I have a bachelor's in women's studies and sociology. Most of the counselors here have at least a bachelor's degree.

What path did you take to get to the job you are in today?

I started out working in domestic violence centers and rape crisis centers, and later I worked as a drug and alcohol counselor in the public schools. While I loved working with kids, I felt I was ready for something that would be less emotional and stressful. I started at the helpline as a counselor working part-time in the evenings, after my day job for the schools. I was promoted to supervisor 6 months later. After working as a supervisor for several years, I left for a while to start my own business in a different industry. But I missed feeling like I was helping people every day, and I'm now enjoying working as a counselor again.

Where might you go from here, if you wanted to advance your career?

One option is to be a supervisor again, either here or in a similar organization. My skills would also transfer to other positions involving counseling or case management, and to many other jobs in the "helping" professions.

What is the worst or most challenging part of your job?

The repetition can be a challenge. On busy days, the calls start to blur together after awhile. Another thing that can be hard is sometimes

Continued

we work with clients in very sad situations. You have to be careful not to take on the callers' feelings of hopelessness.

What is the best part?

I love the work environment. We're all working toward the same common goal—to help people quit. We get a lot of support from one another in weekly meetings and one-on-one. I enjoy counseling because I'm really interested in people, in their lives.

What advice do you have for someone who is interested in your career?

I got here by following my interests and doing the type of work I felt was right for me. I would say do what's most rewarding to you, and look for work that provides an opportunity for personal growth. That's how I've found satisfaction in my career.

BEHAVIORAL SCIENTIST

Job Description

Behavioral scientists study what makes people do the things we do. In public health, they study why people make good and bad choices about food, smoking, safe sex, wearing seatbelts, and many other behaviors. They design and carry out research to find out what helps people make healthy choices or cut down on risky behaviors. Behavioral scientists can be directly involved in community-level studies, or they may concentrate on examining data from local or national surveys to look for patterns. Some are primarily interested in research, while others create public health interventions. They can also be found helping the teams that design campaigns to promote health and prevent disease, and offering guidance on behavioral issues. Hours tend to be reasonable, although projects may sometimes require long hours or weekend work.

Education and Certification

Behavioral scientists usually have doctoral-level degrees in subjects having to do with human behavior, such as psychology, sociology, or anthropology. Some are medical doctors with an interest in human behavior and training in research methods and application. Some are nurses or social workers, often with a PhD in addition to their clinical training.

Core Competencies and Skills

- Initiative and perseverance
- Interest in what makes people tick
- Ability to work as part of a team
- Appreciation of cultural differences
- Tendency to think logically, objectively, and methodically
- Ability to address problems for which solutions have not yet been found
- Understanding of statistics and data analysis (necessary level of expertise varies)

Compensation

The Bureau of Labor Statistics has calculated average salaries for certain social scientists. The median salary for sociologists, for example, is $69,000, with most earning between $41,000 and $122,000. This includes people doing many different types of work, not just public health. Psychology professors have a similar range, with most earning $35,000 to $113,000. Upper-level behavioral scientists at the CDC can earn in the range of $115,000 to $150,000 per year.

Workplaces

Behavioral scientists are found in government agencies, academic institutions, and nonprofit organizations. Private companies also hire behavioral scientists, either to carry out public health projects funded by the government or nonprofits or to work on for-profit efforts that are intended to earn money while addressing health concerns.

Employment Outlook

Overall, employment opportunities for sociologists and anthropologists are expected to increase. However, there are no national statistics for behavioral scientists working in public health. Academic and research positions can be quite competitive, in general, but a growing interest in systems-level health promotion may lead to new opportunities.

For Further Information

Behavioral scientists tend to belong to the associations for their specific fields, such as psychology, psychiatry, or anthropology:

- American Psychological Association (APA)
  www.apa.org
- American Sociological Association (ASA)
  www.asanet.org
- Society for Medical Anthropology (SMA)
  www.medanthro.net

STUDY COORDINATOR

Job Description

Public health research studies are usually originated by professors or doctoral-level researchers. But it's the study coordinators who keep these studies going from day to day. They arrange for recruitment of research participants, set up appointments, manage the data, help prepare updates for funders, and supervise staff. If there are samples or other physical materials involved, they make sure they are properly catalogued and stored. They manage communications, serving as a link between the primary researcher and various assistants, technicians, and clinical or laboratory personnel. Sometimes the coordinator also helps carry out the research. Research coordinators may have opportunities to help author scientific papers and other publications. They may also be involved in submitting grant proposals and obtaining approval from their organizations' Institutional Review Boards, which judge studies for ethical acceptability.

Education and Certification

The educational requirements for this job vary widely. A typical requirement is a bachelor's degree in a field related to the research topic, with training in research principles. Some studies require the coordinator to have a master's degree. If there are clinical responsibilities involved, the coordinator may need to be a nurse or physician assistant. The coordinator of a clinical trial—such as a test of a new medication—may need certification as a Certified Clinical Research Coordinator or Certified Clinical Research Professional; however, these studies are less likely to be considered public health research.

Core Competencies and Skills

- Attention to detail
- Good communication skills
- Excellent organizational skills
- Ability to multitask, prioritize, and delegate tasks efficiently
- Ability to follow directions and use good judgment when unexpected situations arise
- Understanding of research practices, study design, and research ethics
- Knowledge of regulations regarding research

Compensation

Compensation is influenced by the size of the study, whether the coordinator oversees more than one study, the level of responsibility, and the specific tasks involved. A job at one university in the North-Central U.S. requires a master's degree and offers a minimum salary of $30,000 per year. Another, in the Midwest, asks for at least a bachelor's and 2 years' experience and offers $37,000 to $49,000. One example from a major urban area offers $50,000 to $60,000 to start.

Workplaces

Research coordinators involved in public health research work at universities and government agencies; there are also nonprofits and consulting firms that carry out studies.

Employment Outlook

Research is what drives schools of public health, and there is always more to be learned. National data are not available for this specific job title; however, as long as there is funding for research, these jobs should continue to be available. Study coordinator is often a step on the path to a research career or to other opportunities.

For Further Information

■ A good place to learn about public health research projects is at the annual meeting of APHA. Brief research reports from past years' meetings are available at www.apha.org.

REFERENCES

American Diabetes Association. *Diabetes statistics, 2007.* Retrieved from http://www.diabetes.org/diabetes-basics/diabetes-statistics

Centers for Disease Control and Prevention. Chronic disease and health promotion Web site. Retrieved from http://www.cdc.gov/chronicdisease/index.htm

Centers for Disease Control and Prevention. *FastStats: Asthma.* Retrieved from http://www.cdc.gov/nchs/fastats/asthma.htm

Centers for Disease Control and Prevention. *FastStats: Oral health.* Retrieved from http://www.cdc.gov/nchs/FASTATS/dental.htm

Centers for Disease Control and Prevention. *U.S. physical activity statistics, 2007.* Retrieved from http://www.cdc.gov/nccdphp/dnpa/physical/stats/index.htm

6 Public Safety

Public safety intersects with public health in a number of ways. There are nearly five million emergency room visits due to motor vehicle injuries each year. Seat belt and car seat use, drunk driving, drowsy driving, and the safety of teenage drivers are all subjects of public health programs. Public health also addresses playground injuries, drownings and other water-related injuries, sports-related injuries, falls among older adults, and even dog bites. Current thinking is that "accident" isn't really the right word for these events: most "accidents" can be prevented with the right engineering, education, and enforcement of safety laws and regulations.

The prevention of violence is another focus of modern public health. Dating violence, child abuse, elder abuse, domestic violence, and suicide all fall under the topic of violence prevention.

In many areas, emergency medical services (EMS) are also considered part of public health. Over the years, emergency response has grown from simply transport to the hospital to a sophisticated system of pre-hospital care designed to improve survival and minimize disability. EMS systems include dispatchers, ambulance and helicopter services, emergency medical technicians and paramedics, and the emergency rooms and trauma centers where patients are brought for care.

More information is available at the Injury Control and Emergency Health Services section of the APHA Web site (www.apha.org). Other careers that can address safety and injury prevention include epidemiologist, medical epidemiologist, public health nurse, medical officer, health educator, behavioral scientist, and community health worker.

INJURY PREVENTION SPECIALIST

Job Description

Injury prevention specialists assess safety problems in communities, determine the leading causes of serious injuries, and then work on outreach, education, and policy changes that will help. They collect data from sources such as hospitals, clinics, and death certificates. They track motor vehicle accidents, assaults, falls, and other events that could cause disability or death. When the best intervention is already known, they tailor those techniques to the local community; otherwise, they devise their own interventions based on the best available evidence. They look for ways to educate the public, to change the environment to reduce the likelihood of injury, and to enforce rules that promote safety. For example, an injury prevention specialist may run a car seat program with classes for new parents and the provision of free or low-cost car seats, while advocating for stronger laws to promote car seat use. An injury prevention specialist may work directly with the community or may coordinate prevention efforts.

Education and Certification

There is no single education requirement for this career. Some employers look for a degree in environmental health, public health, epidemiology, health education, or another related field, and some specialists are nurses with training in injury prevention. An MPH can be helpful. IHS (Indian Health Service) has an injury prevention training program that is open to non-IHS personnel.

Core Competencies and Skills

- Good communication, presentation, and teaching skills
- Ability to make decisions independently
- Interest in learning how and why specific types of accidents occur
- Understanding of personal and cultural differences that can influence responses to safety efforts

- Knowledge of epidemiology and methods of data analysis
- Understanding of local laws related to injury prevention
- Skills in evidence-based program design and evaluation

Compensation

Differences in responsibilities, educational requirements, and settings make it difficult to give an average salary. State salary data and recent advertisements for injury prevention specialists show salaries from about $35,000 to $70,000 per year, with some program directors earning around $80,000. Salaries can be greater for those with extensive experience and high levels of responsibility.

Workplaces

Injury prevention specialists work for local, state, and federal agencies and for nonprofit organizations. Some hospitals have their own injury prevention centers. Nonprofits often have specific interests such as child safety, water-related injuries, or drunk driving. The military employs injury prevention specialists, both to address everyday injuries and to track combat-related injuries so that protective measures can be optimized.

Employment Outlook

The field of injury prevention has been gradually expanding in recent years. At present, jobs often combine injury prevention and other responsibilities, but as the issue gains prominence, more opportunities specific to injury prevention may become available.

For Further Information

- American Public Health Association—Injury Control and Emergency Health Services Section
  www.apha.org/member groups/sections/aphasections/icehs
- State and Territorial Injury Prevention Directors Association (STIPDA)
  www.stipda.org
- National Center for Injury Prevention and Control
  www.cdc.gov/injury/index.html

DIRECTOR OF EMERGENCY MEDICAL SERVICES

Job Description

The EMS system includes government agencies at the local, regional, state, and even national levels. At each level, there are EMS directors or chiefs who are responsible for making sure the system works effectively. On the local level, many cities and small towns have EMS directors who supervise personnel, handle scheduling, and verify that all workers have the proper certifications. At the county level, EMS agencies oversee the work of smaller local departments and set and enforce policies and regulations. State agencies certify EMS personnel and handle statewide coordination and regulation of EMS.

Typical responsibilities for EMS directors include making decisions about spending, reviewing personnel or departments, ensuring that training and safety programs are in place, and coordinating with the leaders of other emergency services including the fire department (if separate from EMS) and nearby EMS systems. The director also must ensure that the department, its various elements, and any contractors all comply with local, state, and national laws and regulations. EMS directors make decisions about purchasing ambulances or hiring ambulance companies; work with hospitals to ensure high-quality emergency care; and plan for emergencies such as natural disasters or attacks. Policy development is another big part of the job, especially at higher levels.

Running an EMS system is essentially an office job. Some directors who are trained as emergency responders also respond to emergency calls, but as the administrative responsibilities become more complex, this may not be an option.

Education and Certification

An EMS director is usually an experienced manager who has risen through the ranks, either locally or elsewhere. Depending on the specific job, it may be necessary to be certified as a paramedic or licensed as a nurse. Some local jobs require additional emergency-response certifications or even firefighting skills. However, many EMS administrators are not paramedics, firefighters, or emergency medical technicians. Especially at higher levels, the director needs a strong understanding of public policy, administration, and how medical systems are run. Degree requirements vary, but large city or county systems may ask for at least a bachelor's degree in public administration or a business-related field, with a master's degree preferred.

Core Competencies and Skills

- Ability to remain calm under pressure
- Ability to handle multiple tasks and responsibilities at once
- Excellent interpersonal skills
- Strong management ability and financial skills
- Good political and negotiating skills
- Patience with politics and red tape
- Ability to understand and interpret data
- Knowledge of EMS systems and of related local, state, and national laws and regulations

Compensation

Compensation varies greatly, but a salary in the range of $50,000 to $80,000 per year for a city or county EMS director is not uncommon. The director of EMS for a large county or metropolitan area can earn more than $100,000 per year, although most salaries are not this high.

Workplaces

EMS directors work for cities, counties, states, and the military, and there are also opportunities to shape EMS services at the federal level. EMS may be part of the health department or the public safety department, it may be run by or affiliated with the fire department, or it may be a separate agency. There are also director or coordinator roles at ambulance companies and medical centers.

Employment Outlook

There are often jobs available at the local level, although finding an opening in a specific location may be a challenge. Top jobs at the county and state levels are limited and open only to those with strong experience and credentials. However, there are many administrative positions within EMS, particularly in larger systems, which can serve as stepping-stones toward jobs with high levels of responsibility.

For Further Information

- National Association of State EMS Officials (NASEMSO) *www.nasemsd.org*
- National EMS Management Association (NEMSMA) *www.nemsma.org*

PUBLIC HEALTH PROFILE: EMS Director
Virginia Hastings
Executive Director
Inland Counties EMS Agency, San Bernardino, CA

Describe the sort of work you do.

I am in charge of planning, implementation, monitoring, and evaluation for an EMS system that serves three counties in California. That includes overseeing the delivery of paramedic services and the integration of emergency departments and specialty hospitals, such as trauma hospitals or cardiac hospitals. It also includes monitoring and evaluating services to make sure that patients are receiving good care. Another of my department's roles is to ensure compliance with regulations and laws.

What is a typical day like at your job?

I check my emails first thing. I follow up on quick phone calls. I check what assignments I've given others, and I look through my mail. Then, I'll generally have meetings all day long. I attend all the regular meetings of the key county groups—the fire department association, the hospital association, the nurses' association. We discuss contracts and criteria, and then I assign staff members to formulate policies on the things we've talked about. On Tuesdays I go to Board of Supervisors meetings, so a good portion of that day is spent with the elected board members, explaining why I want to approve something.

My job involves a lot of talking and consensus-building. I could sit down right now and put out a directive to say, "You shall do this." But if you don't take the time to build relationships, you can write all the policies you want and they won't be followed.

Continued

My responsibilities also include reviewing my staff members' work. And I do "ride-alongs" with the ambulances and the fire companies to make sure that I keep a "street" feel, because sometimes what you put on paper sounds good but doesn't apply to the real world.

What education or training do you have? Is it typical for your job?

Because this is a government position with a health emphasis, it is helpful to have an education that covers public administration and health care administration. I have a bachelor's degree in public administration and a master's degree in health care administration. Lately, I have been noticing that newer people coming in tend to have worked as paramedics or ER nurses. Those of us who started earlier came up through administrative channels, but the newer people have a field background. I think either type of background could be appropriate for this job.

What path did you take to get to the job you are in today?

I obtained my very first job while I was still in high school. I started as a medical stenographer. When I came to the EMS agency, I knew nothing about EMS My title was Staff Assistant II, and my very first assignment was to analyze a consultant's report dealing with what kind of ambulance service there should be. Later, I became the administrator of the paramedic training institute at Harbor-UCLA Medical Center. I continued to move into jobs with more responsibility until I reached the position of Director of the Los Angeles County EMS Agency. After I retired, I was approached personally by a colleague to apply for my current job. I thought I'd give this a try for a year or so—and that was 5 years ago.

Where might you go from here if you wanted to advance your career?

With the experience I have, I could join a think tank organization dealing with EMS or homeland security. I could also become a consultant, which is a financially rewarding opportunity. In my personal

Continued

goals, I am considering law school because I have become intensely interested in legal issues and legislation related to EMS and health.

What is the worst or most challenging part of your job?

There are sectors that have far more access to local, state, and federal lawmakers than do civil servants like myself. This includes unions that often appear to set policy through powerful legislative contacts. It can be frustrating when policy does not match what I believe would be best for the system.

What is the best part?

I can see the fruits of my labors every time a fire engine, ambulance, or air ambulance is responding, and each time a critically injured person is rushed into surgery at a designated trauma hospital. I know my efforts are worthwhile.

What advice would you give to someone contemplating a career like yours?

Pursue it. It is exciting and it makes a difference. Pursue education in governmental structure; all our programs come under some federal, state, county, or city statute or regulation. It is also important to understand the different cultures of the various entities involved in an EMS system. You can use the strengths of these cultures as you forge public policy.

SPECIALIST IN POISON INFORMATION

Job Description

Specialists in Poison Information (SPIs) educate consumers and health care providers about potential poisons and about what to do if a poisoning occurs. SPIs have to know about common poisons, and they have to know how to obtain information quickly about more than one million different drugs, pesticides, chemicals, and even plants. They use specialized on-line databases, textbooks, and medical journals, and they consult with toxicologists when necessary. Examples from a typical day might include reassuring someone who accidentally took an extra dose of medicine, helping a father whose child swallowed a household cleaning solution, and advising a doctor who is treating a patient who attempted suicide. SPIs also have to be prepared to deal with chemical spills, snake bites, bee stings, and even calls about possible terrorist attacks.

Some SPIs create informational materials, lead training sessions for other health care professionals, and assist with outreach at schools, businesses, and other community sites. They're also part of broader public health efforts. The data they collect go into a national surveillance system that is used to monitor trends in poisonings, track outcomes, and provide early alerts about problems with prescription drugs. Many poison centers have started to work with local health departments in other ways, such as answering after-hours calls to the health department or helping to disseminate information about an epidemic. Some SPIs are also involved in doing original research. Poison control hotlines are active 24 hours a day, 365 days a year, and SPIs generally work 8-, 10-, or 12-hour shifts.

Education and Certification

SPIs are usually registered nurses or pharmacists with special knowledge of toxicology, which can be obtained through on-the-job training at a poison control center. Some are physicians, nurse practitioners, or physician assistants. In most cases, they must earn the credential of Certified Specialist in Poison Information (CSPI), which is provided by the American Association of Poison Control Centers, with recertification every 7 years. For nurses, a current license to practice is essential, and prior clinical experience is helpful and may be expected; some centers prefer nurses who have worked in emergency rooms or intensive care units.

Core Competencies and Skills

- Knack for staying calm under pressure and for keeping others calm as well
- Patience and the ability to listen
- Ability to handle multiple tasks at once
- Ability to communicate effectively with people of different backgrounds and educational levels

- Strong research skills, including the ability to use a computer database and to absorb information rapidly
- Good math skills, for calculating doses, estimating blood levels, and interpreting medical information
- Talent for interviewing, to take an accurate, detailed medical history

Compensation

Salaries vary from center to center. Many centers hire primarily nurses, in part because pharmacists can command higher salaries. Typical salaries for nurse SPIs range from about $40,000 to $90,000.

Workplaces

Poison control centers may be independent nonprofits, or they may be associated with medical centers or health departments.

Employment Outlook

According to a 2008 study in the journal *Clinical Toxicology*, many of the workers at poison control centers are in their 40s or older, suggesting that there will be a need for more specialists as current workers move on or retire. The availability of jobs depends in part on centers' funding and also on the economy as a whole. With nurses and pharmacists expected to be in demand in the next several years, and with so many different opportunities available, it is likely that poison control jobs will remain obtainable for those who are interested. Willingness to begin with a less desirable shift, such as overnight, may be an advantage. Remember, however, that there are only about 60 poison control centers nationwide. Not every city has one, and some cover multiple states.

For Further Information

- American Association of Poison Control Centers (AAPCC)
  www.aapcc.org
- American Academy of Clinical Toxicology (AACT)
  www.clintox.org

PUBLIC HEALTH PROFILE: Specialist in Poison Information
Jean Lubbert, RN, CSPI
Nebraska Regional Poison Center, Omaha, NE

Describe the sort of work you do.

I've worked at the poison center for 23 years. We respond to calls from the public and health care providers about poisonings 24/7. That's our primary role, and it's my main job. The phones always come first. In recent years, we have become more involved with public health issues. Our center also handles calls that come in to the health department about issues like rabies or a potential meningitis outbreak, and we deal with health alerts that come through the CDC.

What is a typical day like at your job?

We have eight incoming phone lines and usually more than one nurse on duty. If I'm doing a morning shift, the night nurse will discuss cases that need further follow up. There could be one, or there could be eight. This involves home follow up as well as health care call backs. I'll look through the database to see if there's anything I should be aware of. And then I'll put my headphones on, and off I go. As each call comes in, I obtain a very detailed history, check my references as needed, and enter notes into the computer. I determine how toxic the exposure is and provide detailed recommendations. I need to communicate in a way that each caller can understand. If it is a parent, I'll talk to them differently than I would to a health care provider.

If it turns out to be a nontoxic substance I don't need to follow up with the caller, but if it is gasoline, for example, we do a 1-hour and a 4-hour call-back to verify no chemical aspiration has occurred. If I'm not certain about what to do for a particular case, I check with other professionals. There is always a board-certified toxicologist on call for further input depending on the complexity of the case.

If there's downtime on the phones there are many other things to work on. Sometimes health care providers want a copy of our protocols or an article from our files, so we'll fax them. Quality

Continued

assurance is important, so I may be auditing cases, reading abstracts, or reviewing primary literature to assist with writing protocols. Sometimes I'm scheduled to work on research. We also have pharmacy students and emergency room residents who do rotations here. It adds variety to our job, because we can be mentors and we always work as a team.

What education or training do you have? Is it typical for your job?

Most CSPIs are registered nurses or registered pharmacists. I went to a liberal arts college for 1 year after high school, and then I went to the University of Nebraska Medical Center College of Nursing for an associate's degree nursing program. I have taken classes toward obtaining my bachelor's degree. After working 2 years or taking the equivalent of 2,000 calls, I sat for the national certification examination to become a CSPI.

What path did you take to get to the job you are in today?

I was working as a nurse in a hospital. I worked 3 years in neurosurgery and 2 years in the adult intensive care unit (ICU). And then I saw an ad in the paper for a poison center specialist, and it really intrigued me. Poison center work was nothing I had learned about in nursing school. The managing director was happy to hear that I had ICU experience. That nursing experience has helped me immensely in my work here.

Where might you go from here, if you wanted to advance your career?

For myself personally, I like the combination of the things we do here. I find the variety of work challenging and rewarding. For someone who wanted to try a different job, the skills would likely translate to certain aspects of public health nursing—like how to collect and interpret data. Critical thinking and communication skills are huge benefits if you were to work in another type of telephone triage service.

Continued

What is the worst or most challenging part of your job?

If you're super busy and you've got multiple lines going, you need to prioritize. And sometimes you have difficult callers. They're saying, "Somebody poisoned me," but it could really be a mental health issue. Staying calm, efficient, and precise in recommendations gives the best patient outcome.

What is the best part?

Even though you don't see the patient or the health care provider you're talking to, people are often really grateful that you are helping them. Not only that, but you never stop learning in this job. It is so rewarding.

What advice do you have for someone who is interested in your career?

You have to have good communication skills, you have to be empathetic, and you have to have good listening skills. If you want to help people, it's a great job to have!

FORENSIC PATHOLOGIST

Job Description

A forensic pathologist is a physician who assists with death investigations, often through a city, county, or state medical examiner's office or in affiliation with an elected lay coroner's office. The job varies by state, but the medical examiner is typically involved in investigating cases of sudden, unexpected death; death from accidental injury, violence, or poisoning; deaths outside of a hospital or hospice setting; deaths of infants and children; deaths in correctional institutions and state mental health facilities; deaths of people in police custody; and any other unusual case. When an autopsy is needed, the job goes to a forensic pathologist. These experts use knowledge of medicine, toxicology, criminalistics, and evidence collection and processing to provide information for police investigations, and when necessary they provide courtroom testimony.

In addition, forensic pathologists serve the cause of public health by watching for trends that could indicate a disease outbreak, the emergence of a new infectious disease, or a bioterrorism attack. Their reports contribute to surveillance for child mortality, intimate partner homicide, deaths due to drug abuse, and other types of deaths that public health programs may be able to address. Some also practice clinical forensic pathology, which means examining living patients for evidence of a crime such as rape or child abuse. The job can also include working with local hospitals on quality assurance for trauma and emergency care, collaborating with other agencies to review child fatalities, tracking trends in drug abuse, and participating in programs to promote driver safety.

Education and Certification

A forensic pathologist must have an MD or DO degree, and must have completed residency training in anatomic pathology, or anatomic and clinical pathology, plus a fellowship in forensic pathology. Certification by the American Board of Pathology, which requires an examination and ongoing education, is often expected.

Core Competencies and Skills

- Ability to handle unpleasant sights and smells without becoming ill or upset
- Tendency to ask questions and seek answers that are as complete as possible
- Attention to detail
- Thorough understanding of human anatomy
- Knowledge of toxicology, pathology, ballistics, infectious and chronic disease, and other subjects related to potential causes of death
- Knowledge of laws and procedures for the collection of evidence

Compensation

Salaries vary by location and responsibility. Typical salaries offered for forensic pathologists range from the low $100,000s to the low $200,000s. Chief Medical Examiners and those who consult for coroners can earn quite a bit more.

Workplaces

In some places, the office of the medical examiner is part of the health department. In others, it is a separate part of city, county, or state government. Some areas have only coroners and no medical examiner's office at all; in those jurisdictions, forensic pathologists are hired as consultants on a case-by-case basis. Forensic pathologists also work for hospitals or private medical groups that contract with the local government to provide forensic autopsy services.

Employment Outlook

The need for pathologists in general is expected to be strong over the next few years. With only about 600 board-certified forensic pathologists currently in full-time practice, the job opportunities in this specialty should be good. There has been discussion of converting the existing coroner systems to medical examiner systems within the next decade or two; if this happens, there may be many additional job openings.

For Further Information

- College of American Pathologists (CAP)
  www.cap.org
- National Association of Medical Examiners (NAME)
  thename.org
- American Academy of Forensic Sciences (AAFS)
  www.aafs.org

REFERENCE

Centers for Disease Control and Prevention. National Center for Injury Prevention and Control Web site. Retrieved from http://www.cdc.gov/injury

7   Maternal and Child Health

Maternal and child health is a major area of public health. More than half of American women who give birth receive services through programs administered by the Maternal and Child Health Bureau (MCHB). Millions of women, infants, and children receive nutritional support through a program at the USDA. There are numerous federal, state, and local programs addressing infant mortality, birth defects, and access to prenatal care.

Some maternal and child health efforts apply to everyone, such as newborn screenings to test for certain congenital disorders and hearing ability. Other programs focus on specific populations: teenage mothers, children with developmental delay, and low-income families. There are programs to address perinatal depression, encourage breastfeeding, raise immunization rates, increase the number of children receiving health care services, provide family planning services, reduce the risk of sudden infant death syndrome, and teach parenting skills. A national monitoring system is gathering data to try to discover why some babies are born healthy and some are not. In addition to programs run by government agencies, there are many nonprofits dedicated to issues in maternal and child health.

Many people working in this area belong to the APHA section on Maternal and Child Health (http://www.apha.org/membergroups/sections/aphasections/mch). The APHA section on Population,

Reproductive, and Sexual Health includes family planning issues (http://www.apha.org/membergroups/sections/aphasections/population).

There are many different opportunities in maternal and child health; this chapter outlines just a few. Also see the descriptions for public health social worker, nutritionist, health teacher, injury prevention specialist, and director/officer of minority health.

DEPUTY DIRECTOR/FAMILY HEALTH SERVICES

Job Description

Each state has a department dedicated to public health services for parents, children, and teens. These departments have various names— family health services; maternal and child health services; maternal, child, and adolescent health; and so on. The deputy director typically is the administrator who oversees the finances, handles personnel issues, guides the daily work of the department, and assists the director with decision making and long range planning.

These departments house programs such as registries of birth defects, newborn screening systems, programs to track and prevent child abuse, educational programs to reduce teen pregnancies, family planning services, nutrition services, and more. Each of these sections has its own coordinator, but the department administrator makes sure that they are meeting goals, staying within their budgets, and identifying and addressing both new and ongoing needs. When there are changes in the budget, the deputy director helps determine what services must be cut and which should be preserved. He also helps program coordinators write grant proposals, participates in personnel decisions, and works with clinical staff to make sure that patients at community clinics receive appropriate care. This is largely a desk job, but there may also be opportunities to go out into the community and observe the department's programs in action.

Education and Certification

This position requires substantial experience with administration, as well as with the programs within the department. An MPH is particularly useful, because it provides a good understanding of maternal and child health issues. An MPA can also be a good fit, with experience or other training in public health. Some people in this role have clinical training, such as a nursing degree.

Core Competencies and Skills

- Strong management and financial skills
- Excellent written and spoken communication skills
- Good planning skills, including the ability to break large projects down into specific tasks
- Knowledge of health issues that are of particular relevance to parents and children
- Knowledge of state and federal requirements for health and social services programs
- Ability to understand statistical and epidemiologic data
- Experience managing a public health program

Compensation

Salaries depend on the local cost of living, amount of experience, and pay structure within the health department. In one state with a relatively low cost of living, for example, a typical salary would be in the range of $70,000 to the mid-$90,000s.

Workplaces

This is usually a state government job, but some city and county health departments also have sections dedicated to maternal, child, and family health. County-level programs tend to focus more on public health nursing programs, such as home visits and clinic services.

Employment Outlook

There is generally just one job at this level in family health services for each state. However, there are many administrative opportunities within maternal, child, and family health departments. Individual programs may each have their own managers, there may be directors who oversee multiple areas within the department, and programs may be divided up among different areas of the state. Specific requirements for these jobs, such as an MPH or a clinical degree, vary by department.

For Further Information

■ Association of Maternal and Child Health Programs (AMCHP) *www.amchp.org*

PUBLIC HEALTH PROFILE: Deputy Director/Family Health Services
Chris Haag, MPH

Deputy Director, Bureau of Family Health Services
Alabama Department of Public Health, Montgomery, AL

Describe the sort of work you do.

I oversee the finances, administration, and program operations for the Alabama Bureau of Family Health Services. My responsibilities include applying for grants, working on protocols and procedural issues, overseeing the budget, and finding new ways to address specific public health problems. Part of my job is knowing when the time is right to tackle certain issues. When divisions within the bureau propose new projects and programs, I guide them in making strategic decisions. I make sure that the budget includes everything that's essential, I ask if other states have done similar programs and what they cost, and I consider whether it makes more sense to create a new system in-house or to purchase an outside product or service.

What is a typical day like at your job?

I have lots of meetings. Today, there were several meetings on finance. Budgets are being reduced, but people still need public health services, and we have to figure out how to do more with less. I also met this morning with some staff from our child health program. We're launching an online system for our newborn screening program. We walked through what we need to do, what the timeline is, and what it will cost.

When we need approval for a new program or service, I keep track of who is responsible, what has been done, and what needs to be done. I coordinate strategy with my boss, and with the staff who will work with state leaders to get approval and funding. I frequently

Continued

receive proposed legislation to read, and I provide comments on the potential impact. Personnel management also consumes much of my time.

What education or training do you have? Is it typical for your job?

I have an MPH and a bachelor's degree in education. The training you get with an MPH is very helpful for this job.

What path did you take to get to the job you are in today?

My first public health job was as a health educator at a county health department. When I moved to Montgomery, I continued working as a health educator, this time with the state health department. Then I spent 4 years as the bureau administrator here, mostly handling the finances. I never really liked that job, but I learned a lot from it. And then the deputy director position opened up, and I decided to interview for it.

Where might you go from here, if you wanted to advance your career?

I'm happy where I am. For me, the next thing may be to earn a doctorate in public administration. In Alabama, currently the Director of the Bureau of Family Services must be a medical doctor, so I couldn't be promoted into that position. Staff assistant to the State Health Officer might be a next step, but being promoted into that position is very difficult and I am not sure I would be interested in that level work. I enjoy what I do now.

What is the worst or most challenging part of your job?

Having to lay people off is the worst. When funding decreases, we have to identify services or programs we can cut. A close second is firing someone. It can also be challenging to deal with politics. My team and I have to craft solutions that work politically but at the same time meet very real needs.

Continued

What is the best part?

I like going out into the community. It is a chance to see how what we do is helping an individual kid or a family. At times, I can even help directly. If a family can't afford the special foods for a child with a metabolic disorder, sometimes we can develop a more reasonable fee agreement which lets families buy the foods at a lower cost.

What advice do you have for someone who is interested in your career?

If you want to work your way up to a leadership position, worry less about what your job description is and more about doing what's needed. I got to where I am because my boss knows that whatever he asks for, I'll give it 100%. I will figure it out and get it done.

HOME VISIT NURSE

Job Description

There are several public health programs that involve home visits by nurses, not to provide traditional nursing care, but to help catch problems and increase the potential for good health. For example, a home visit nurse might spend an hour or two each week teaching a teenage mother life skills (changing and feeding the baby, checking for safety hazards, etc.) that will help her to be a good parent. She makes sure that baby's development is on track, and if there is a problem, she connects the mother with services that can help. She helps mothers access other services, too, from housing to general educational development (GED) programs to domestic violence hotlines. The home visit nurse might also provide counseling to a teenage parent who is struggling with drugs, alcohol, or mental health problems. Some programs provide continued home visits through the child's early years.

In addition to working with clients, home visit nurses also have to maintain patient charts and keep up with new regulations, requirements, and research. The job may include some evening and weekend visits.

Education and Certification

A home visit nurse must have a current state registered nurse (RN) license. A BSN degree (as opposed to a nursing diploma or associate's degree) may be required. Home visiting experience, training in obstetrics and prenatal care, and experience as a pediatric nurse can all be helpful. Once a nurse is hired for a home visit program, there is usually a period of on-the-job training, as well.

Core Competencies and Skills

- Flexibility and patience to deal with missed appointments, traffic, and challenging patients
- Willingness to travel to low-income, potentially dangerous areas
- Strong initiative and organizational skills
- Knack for teaching and for helping people set and meet goals
- Appreciation of diverse cultures and ways of thinking
- Knowledge of or an interest in learning about pediatric development, parenting skills, and basic mental health care
- Knowledge of local, state, and national programs to assist parents and families
- Fluency in a language other than English (may be needed)

Compensation

In one major city, home visit nurses in a public health program earn from the $60,000s to over $75,000. In a southern state with a lower cost of living, nurses in a similar program start at about $45,000.

Workplaces

Home visit nurses often work for health departments. They also work for nonprofit organizations and for private companies that contract with public health programs. In addition to maternal and child health programs, nurses who make home visits can also be found in outreach programs for the elderly.

Employment Outlook

One of the most prominent home visit programs has been going strong for more than 30 years, and a track record of good outcomes means that programs are likely to continue. Competition for jobs varies, but some programs have actually found it a challenge to recruit nurses, since this work is quite different from a typical nursing role.

For Further Information

- Visiting Nurse Associations of America (VNAA)
  vnaa.org
- Also see the organizations listed with the Public Health Nurse job description.

COMMUNITY HEALTH WORKER

Job Description

Community health workers (CHWs) go out into neighborhoods, housing projects, barber shops, and other community settings to work directly with populations in need. They are usually members of the communities they serve. CHWs provide health education and can assist with access to care, but they are not licensed health care providers. Instead, their primary role is as a link between underserved communities, where people are often suspicious of government and doctors, and the health service mainstream. Through individual visits, presentations to community groups, and the distribution of written information, CHWs can provide education on many important health issues.

In some maternal and child health programs, CHWs work directly with pregnant women who are at risk of poor birth outcomes. They do outreach to locate these women and interest them in the program, help them find prenatal care services, encourage them to make and keep appointments, provide basic education on health issues, and help them find resources such as GED programs and safe childcare. CHWs are trained to be sensitive to issues such as poverty or violence that might serve as barriers to good health.

In addition to maternal and child health, CHWs are also used with other health issues and populations. This job has many different titles, including "lay health educator," "peer educator," and "promotor" or "promotora" (used in Spanish-speaking communities).

Education and Certification

Educational expectations vary from a GED to a college degree. CHWs are often trained by their employers for the specific services they will provide. There are also training opportunities at community colleges, local nonprofits, and other health-oriented settings. Some states have specific training and certification requirements.

Core Competencies and Skills

- Patience and a sense of humor
- Outgoing, friendly nature
- Excellent communication skills, including good listening skills
- Ability to help people solve problems, without doing it for them
- Interest in helping build community strength
- Basic understanding of health and health care issues
- Personal understanding of the culture of the community being served
- Ability to be comfortable among different types of people
- Fluency in a language other than English, if needed to communicate with clients

Compensation

A national study of the CHW workforce, completed in 2007, found that about two-thirds of newly hired CHWs earned between minimum wage and $13 per hour (about $25,000 per year for a full-time job). Experienced workers earned more, with many making $15 per hour or above. A 2009 summary from the Community Health Worker Special Primary Interest group at APHA estimates somewhat higher salaries, starting around $35,000 to $42,000, with a rise to $52,000 with experience.

Workplaces

CHWs are employed by local governments, nonprofit organizations, health care facilities, a few public schools, and community health programs based at academic institutions.

Employment Outlook

The idea of using community members to promote health and improve access to care seems to be gaining momentum, so it is likely that job opportunities will increase.

For Further Informations

- The American Association of Community Health Workers is a new organization that, as of this writing, does not yet have a Web site.
- American Public Health Association—CHW Section *www.apha.org/membergroups/sections/aphassections/chw*
- Center for Sustainable Health Outreach *www.usm.edu/csho*

WIC NUTRITIONIST

Job Description

The national Special Supplemental Nutrition Program for Women, Infants, and Children (WIC) is a long-running federal program that provides supplemental foods, nutrition education, and health care referrals for low-income women who are pregnant or have recently given birth, and for infants and young children at risk of poor nutrition. WIC nutritionists determine whether women and children are eligible for the program and provide vouchers for approved foods. The foods WIC supplies were chosen to help meet specific needs in populations at risk of poor nutrition. But WIC nutritionists do more than hand out vouchers. They ask about health problems that could affect nutrition, like food allergies in a child. They check for anemia and monitor children's growth. They educate women about healthy eating and teach them how to make affordable, nutritious meals. They work to combat child obesity. Some WIC programs encourage exercise, help women obtain car seats, or offer cooking demonstrations.

WIC nutritionists have to strike a careful balance between educating women and allowing them to make their own choices, and they have to be sensitive to social and cultural differences. Some clients are eager to learn, while others may be challenging to work with. The job also requires knowledge of program regulations and requirements, which can be quite complex. Some nutritionists have the opportunity to bring additional creativity to the work, such as designing recipes and menu plans or writing a monthly newsletter. A 40-hour workweek is typical, although some programs offer appointments on evenings and weekends.

Education and Certification

Nutritionists and dietitians generally must have at least a bachelor's degree, with a focus on nutrition or a related subject. Specific requirements for WIC nutritionists vary. Often, they must be registered dietitians (RDs), which requires a bachelor's degree, certain courses specific to nutrition, hands-on training, and an examination. Details on the RD credential are available from the Commission on Dietetic Registration at www.cdrnet.org. A master's degree in nutrition is usually required for supervisory work.

Core Competencies and Skills

- Strong communication skills, including both speaking and listening
- Excellent teaching skills
- Flexible thinking, to adapt recommendations to individual clients' lifestyles and needs
- Understanding of local communities, particularly their cultures and food traditions
- Knowledge of WIC regulations and requirements
- Thorough knowledge of nutritional needs during pregnancy, breastfeeding, and early childhood

Compensation

Dietitians and nutritionists in general earn salaries ranging from about $30,000 per year to about $70,000, with about half earning above $50,000. These numbers are typical for WIC nutritionists, as well.

Workplaces

WIC programs employ a large number of nutritionists nationwide. There are WIC programs run by health departments, nonprofit organizations, and hospitals and health centers.

Employment Outlook

WIC is a very large program—serving more than 9 million women, infants, and children—and there are often jobs available. Some programs find that nutritionists stay in their jobs for many years, which may limit the number of openings, but some also report that job openings can be hard to fill.

For Further Information

■ American Dietetic Association (ADA)
www.eatright.org
■ The Public Health/Community Nutrition Practice Group of the ADA
www.phcnpg.org
■ American Public Health Association—Food and Nutrition Section
www.apha.org/membergroups/sections/aphasections/food
■ National WIC Association (NWA)
www.nwica.org

PUBLIC HEALTH PROFILE: WIC Nutritionist
Rosemary Flynn, MS, RD
Public Health Nutritionist
Women, Infants and Children (WIC) Program
Nassau County Health Department, Uniondale, NY

Describe the sort of work you do.

I'm a nutritionist with a WIC program run by a county health department. We give women information about nutrition and help them find ways to stretch their food dollars. We see the women for individual appointments, and we also offer classes on topics like cooking and portion control. We really encourage physical activity, too. In the summer, we connect with farmers markets and give our clients coupons to buy fresh produce. One of our goals is to lay down the groundwork when children are young, so they'll make healthier choices later.

What is a typical day like at your job?

I start by preparing for appointments or classes. When I'm teaching classes, I usually have about four sessions, and I don't have patient

Continued

appointments on those days. On a day with clients, I'll see about 20 women. Visits are scheduled to last 15 minutes each, although sometimes they go over.

At the visits, I measure height and weight and check for anemia, for both mother and child. I ask about physical activity and about television time for the child. We talk about their eating habits, including not just what foods they eat but when and how they have their meals. Once I have that information I can encourage healthy eating habits. I see a lot of overweight children, and many of those moms need guidance on how to make fast food and soda occasional treats instead of everyday things. I ask about substance abuse, conditions at the home, and dental care. At the end of the appointment, I give the woman 3 months of WIC checks.

Appointments don't always go smoothly. Sometimes a woman will come in, and her papers aren't filled out, and the child is crying, and just filling out those papers becomes a big deal. I have to find out what's going on in her life that makes even that first task so difficult. Children present their own challenges. If a child won't eat anything but mashed potatoes, I can't just say, "Have him eat more fruits and vegetables," because he won't! I have to think about getting him better nutrition in ways that he will accept.

What education or training do you have? Is it typical for your job?

I am an RD, licensed by the state as a certified dietitian/nutritionist, and I'm also certified as a lactation consultant. I have both bachelor's and master's degrees in nutrition. Among my colleagues in the WIC program, about half have a master's degree, and supervisors are required to have that level of education.

What path did you take to get to the job you are in today?

I started as a clinical dietitian, working in hospitals. But then I was given an opportunity to take a part-time job doing public health nutrition. I realized I enjoyed that more than my full-time job! I had to

Continued

learn a lot to make the transition to public health, because it is very different working in a community than working at the bedside. After I took some time off to raise my family, I went back to school to earn that master's degree. I thought I'd go back to clinical nutrition, because that's where the money was—but then, while I was looking for a new job, an ad popped up for the WIC program. And I thought, that's what I want to do.

Where might you go from here, if you wanted to advance your career?

The next step for someone at my level might be to oversee a WIC program. We have a nutritionist from the city who comes and audits what we do, and there are state supervisors. If I wanted a really high-level career, I'd have to leave the practice of nutrition. I could aim to become a program director, or I could be involved in selling pharmaceuticals.

What is the worst or most challenging part of your job?

There are some clients who are difficult to deal with. There are a few who are so set in their ways, I know that no matter what I say, their behavior is not going to provide the healthiest environment for the child.

What is the best part?

The best part is when I see someone succeed. It is when a really obese child comes back after 6 months, and he hasn't gained any weight, and he's grown 6 inches. It is rewarding to help a mom know what to do when her child is overdue to graduate from a bottle to a cup, and to see the child finally make that change.

What advice do you have for someone who is interested in your career?

Do an internship first and make sure this is something you really want to do. Then look deep inside yourself, and see if you can be tolerant

Continued

and empathic and compassionate and nonjudgmental. If a woman is sitting in front of you and tells you she wants to terminate a pregnancy, what are you going to do? Or what if she says she's never going to stop smoking cigarettes? You can't bring your own morals and values to these visits. You have to leave them outside the door.

8   Pharmaceuticals and Drug Safety

How do we know that a prescription medicine will actually do what the manufacturer claims? How can we be sure that a bottle labeled "aspirin" actually contains aspirin? And how can we be confident that a medication is more likely to help than to harm? This is the realm of public health professionals concerned with drug evaluation and safety.

The Food and Drug Administration (FDA) oversees regulation of prescription and over-the-counter medicines. The FDA's many responsibilities include not only determining the safety and efficacy of drugs before they can be sold but also regulating advertising, inspecting manufacturers, ensuring accurate labeling, doing ongoing safety monitoring, protecting against counterfeit medicines, and more. The FDA also regulates blood products, vaccines, and other biological products.

There are many opportunities for public health professionals in drug evaluation and safety. Much of this work goes on at the FDA, but there are also opportunities in other government agencies, industry, academia, and the nonprofit world. Other jobs that touch on drug safety include epidemiologist, veterinarian, medical officer, consumer safety officer, and medical epidemiologist.

PHARMACIST

Job Description

Although "public health pharmacist" isn't a widely used term here in the United States, there are plenty of pharmacists helping to promote the health of our population. Some pharmacists combine their pharmacy training with work in policy making, epidemiology, or other areas of public health. They can be involved in analyzing reports about drug side effects and deciding if extra warnings should be added or if the drug should be recalled. They may contribute their specialized knowledge to decisions about new drug regulations or laws. There are public health pharmacists involved in evaluating proposals for new medications, as well.

There are also public health pharmacists performing traditional tasks such as compounding and dispensing drugs. The Indian Health Service (IHS) includes pharmacists in its efforts to protect and improve the health of Native Americans. Some pharmacists are involved in disaster planning. Other roles include managing drugs for rare diseases, studying the safety of dietary supplements, and helping to manage programs that provide medicine for people with HIV/AIDS.

Education and Certification

A pharmacist just finishing training needs a Doctor of Pharmacy (PharmD) degree in order to be licensed. This is a relatively new requirement, so older pharmacists often hold different degrees. Licensure also requires examinations covering drug information and state and federal regulations and laws. Pharmacists who are interested in public health often pursue MPHs, and some pharmacy schools offer combined PharmD/MPH programs. Experience in research and data analysis can be especially helpful. Residency rotations are available at government agencies including the FDA.

Core Competencies and Skills

- Tendency to be detail-oriented
- Aptitude for science and for research
- Ability to break down complex problems into manageable steps
- Ability to see how research and data apply to real-world problems
- Good interpersonal skills, including the ability to communicate with people from other disciplines

- Understanding of statistics and epidemiology (necessary level of knowledge varies)
- Broad knowledge of drugs, how they work, and drug interactions
- Understanding of community dynamics (for pharmacists who will be working in community-level programs)

Compensation

Most pharmacists earn between $77,000 and $130,000 per year. Pharmacists who work for the federal government may earn a little less than those in hospital or retail pharmacies, although government jobs with high levels of responsibility can pay well over $100,000 per year. Pharmacists who work in public health often find that the lifestyle and job satisfaction tend to offset any difference in salary.

Workplaces

In the federal government, the departments within HHS—such as FDA, CDC, and HRSA—employ many pharmacists to work on public health matters. Many public health pharmacists get their start at IHS. There are many opportunities through the USPHS Commissioned Corps. Pharmacists also fill public health-oriented roles at state and local health departments and in the military.

Employment Outlook

The overall outlook for pharmacist jobs is expected to be excellent, with more jobs available than there are pharmacists looking for work. In public health, there will likely be a continued need for pharmacists in drug safety, disaster planning, and public programs. Given the recent interest in quality assurance, medication effectiveness, and cost control, there may be an increasing demand for pharmacists in public health; however, this depends on how the health system evolves.

For Further Information

- APHA may add a specialty section for public health pharmacists.
- Visit university PharmD/MPH programs and government agencies' Web sites including fda.gov
- American Pharmacists' Association
  www.pharmacist.com

PUBLIC HEALTH PROFILE: Pharmacist
Lt. Brian Parker, PharmD
Pharmacist
San Xavier Indian Health Center, Tucson, AZ

Describe the sort of work you do.

I'm a pharmacist with the U.S. Public Health Service Commissioned Corps, assigned to IHS. I work at a clinic on an Indian reservation in Tucson, AZ. Right now, a lot of what I do is similar to what a pharmacist might do at a drugstore. I answer questions from patients, doctors, and nurses. I make sure that medications match the conditions they're prescribed for and that doses are correct. Every 3 or 4 weeks I spend a few days at our hospital, where I perform similar duties. We're also working on drug reconciliation and on polypharmacy—trying to help patients reduce the number of pills they have to take.

What is a typical day like at your job?

On some days I'm primarily doing refills; on others, I'm doing all the new prescriptions or checking prescriptions our technicians have filled. If the dose seems too high or too low, it doesn't seem like the right drug, or it seems like a drug is missing from what's been prescribed, I call up the doctor or nurse and ask. Usually with new prescriptions, I tell the patient a little bit about the medicine. A lot of times they have something they're uncomfortable asking the doctor, so they ask me.

I'm also helping implement an automated refill line, and I've created a pamphlet and posters to help the patients use it. Hopefully, I'll be training soon to participate in our pharmacist-run anticoagulation clinic. Our health center is also looking at having pharmacists perform medication reconciliation, do patient counseling, and look at other laboratory results, too. Together with the doctor we would make adjustments to the patients' drug therapy.

What education or training do you have? Is it typical for your job?

I have a PharmD degree. I originally went to school to be a physical therapist, so I also have a BS in exercise physiology.

Continued

What path did you take to get to the job you are in today?

In the summer during college, I worked at a drug store, and I'd often hand patients their medications. I found out that I liked talking to people. I only needed one more class to qualify for pharmacy school, and I decided to do it. After pharmacy school, I worked for a while as a traveling pharmacist, and I was sent to different areas on short-term assignments. I had always wanted to work on an Indian reservation, so I asked if I could do that. They sent me here for 8 months, and then a permanent job opened up and I was asked to stay. That's when I joined the Commissioned Corps.

Where might you go from here, if you wanted to advance your career?

I'm thinking about getting my MPH and doing EIS, and I also want to get my Board Certified Pharmacotherapy Specialist certification. In the Public Health Service I can get out from behind the counter at the pharmacy, become a deputy director or compliance officer, do epidemiology, serve as chair of a public health organization commit-tee, help with disaster response, work in drug approval at the FDA ... there are so many options!

What is the worst or most challenging part of your job?

I like Arizona, and my primary site's not too remote, but I'm far from my family. Also, because of how my schedule works, some days it's hard to predict what time my workday will end.

What is the best part?

The other pharmacists and our technicians and I really get along well, and we help each other out when there is a lot of work to do. I also like talking to the doctors and hearing if they've seen anything fas-cinating in clinic that day. And I enjoy working with the patients. People will come in with different stories, and I love to talk with them about what's going on in their lives.

Continued

What advice do you have for someone who is interested in your career?

Talk to as many people in the job as you can, in as many areas as you can. I can describe my job, and it sounds wonderful—but someone else might not like it at all. It might be different at another IHS site, so it's worth asking three or four people at different sites. You'll get a better understanding of the pros and the cons.

MEDICAL OFFICER/DRUG EVALUATION AND SAFETY

Job Description

The FDA employs doctors as medical officers to help ensure the safety and effectiveness of prescription and over-the-counter medicines. These physicians interpret research and make important decisions about whether drugs should be approved, how they are manufactured, and what precautions should be in place. Some medical officers are involved in reviewing drug studies. Some make sure that drug labels are accurate. Some inspect manufacturing plants to verify that pills, tablets, and other medicines are being made correctly and are not contaminated. Medical officers also evaluate complaints and reports of side effects from drugs, and they have influence over the creation of new warning labels and even the removal of drugs from the market. The FDA hires doctors for other medical officer roles, too, in areas including food safety, vaccine effectiveness, the safety of blood products and medical devices, and radiation control.

Medical officers generally work standard hours, except when important projects or emergencies require extra time. They may also need to take time outside of work to read medical journals and keep up with the latest research.

Education and Certification

An FDA medical officer must have an MD or DO degree and, usually, must have completed residency training and be licensed to practice. Some medical officer jobs require only 1 year of residency, and the licensure requirement may be waived if there is no direct patient care. There are opportunities for many different types of doctors, but training relevant to the focus of the job is important. For example, a medical officer who evaluates drugs that affect the digestive system would be expected to have expertise in gastroenterology.

Core Competencies and Skills

- Ability to work with people from different fields and backgrounds
- Confidence to make decisions that may be controversial
- Patience with paperwork and red tape
- Understanding of research design and data analysis
- Willingness to read complex and sometimes lengthy documents
- Strong medical background, with an understanding of how the body works and of what happens in disease
- Knowledge of basic pharmacology (essentially, how drugs work)

Compensation

Typical salaries for FDA medical officers are in the range of $85,000 to $130,000 per year, with adjustments for location. Depending on responsibilities and experience, salaries can reach $150,000 or more.

Workplaces

The FDA is the primary federal agency concerned with drug safety and effectiveness. There are also opportunities within industry to help monitor drug safety and ensure compliance with regulations.

Employment Outlook

The work of the FDA is ongoing, and medical officers will continue to play an important role. There are often openings for qualified physicians. Finding a specific job in drug safety may take a while, but there are medical officers in many different areas within the FDA.

For Further Information

- Food and Drug Administration (FDA)
  www.fda.gov

PUBLIC HEALTH PROFILE: Medical Officer
Sandra Kweder, MD
Deputy Director, Office of New Drugs
U.S. Food and Drug Administration, Washington, DC

Continued

Describe the sort of work you do.

My job is to oversee the scientists and public health experts who make decisions about medicines and determine which ones should be available for use. That includes deciding how drugs should be studied and, once they've been studied, if they're safe and effective and eligible for marketing. This includes prescription medicines as well as over-the-counter products like headache or allergy medicines. My department also looks at a drug's role in the marketplace and what patients and prescribers need to know. Once drugs are on the market, we monitor them closely for safety. We are really public health agents at FDA, but we do our job by regulatory oversight of the multi-billion dollar pharmaceutical industry.

What is a typical day like at your job?

When I first started, my job was to review individual clinical studies and think about the details of how a specific drug might go from the laboratory to the bedside. Now, my days are about guiding the overall system we have at the FDA for new drug review. I am making decisions that may affect many drugs and how they are studied or marketed. I oversee other medical officers and scientists. My office has over 900 professionals in it, all of whom are involved with overseeing drug development, clinical trials, and marketing applications. I meet with directors of offices under mine to talk about what they are reviewing in their divisions and what the scientific, public health, and management challenges are, including those related to new findings about the safety of drugs already on the market. I often advise them on how to handle problems that come up.

In between meetings, I try to keep up with about 200 emails a day. Often, those contain something I need to read and approve, such as a position paper, a review, or a press release. I often interact with very senior executives in the pharmaceutical industry, speak to the press, and represent the FDA at academic conferences, consumer and industry group meetings, and Congressional hearings.

Continued

What education or training do you have? Is it typical for your job?

You need to be a doctor, an MD or DO. It helps to have been through residency training and have some clinical experience, so you understand how drugs are used. It is also helpful if you've been involved in doing clinical studies.

What path did you take to get to the job you are in today?

I was fresh out of residency when I started at the FDA, as a medical officer in the anti-virals division. At that time, there was only one drug available to treat HIV, and we were inundated with new drug proposals. We were constantly hiring new people. Pretty soon I was one of the people with the most experience, and I became a team leader. When the job of Director of the Division of Surveillance and Epidemiology opened up, I was asked to fill that role on a temporary basis—and that turned into 2 years. Next I chose to advance my own knowledge with a fellowship in medical complications of pregnancy. When I came back, I worked as deputy director for an office of drug evaluation and then, with more growth and changes within the FDA, I took on the role of acting director of the Office of New Drugs and then became the full-time deputy director.

Where might you go from here, if you wanted to advance your career?

If I wanted to advance, it could be to a job with even more responsibility within the FDA or I could seek a leadership role in another agency or organization. Many with the experience I have had find roles in the pharmaceutical industry or even working with large health care organizations.

What is the worst or most challenging part of your job?

It is hard having to be the bad guy. Sometimes I have to deliver bad news to a company, and I have to be tough on them. Sometimes it is a staff member who needs to improve his or her work. Back when I

Continued

first started as a medical officer, the things I liked least were statistics and chemistry. I was always grateful that I worked with chemists and statisticians who really loved those disciplines and would help me!

What is the best part?

One reason my job is so interesting is that almost no two circumstances are the same. There may be parallels from one drug to another, but there is always something new. There is always a new puzzle, and I am learning all the time.

What advice do you have for someone who is interested in your career?

If you're a physician who likes science, likes puzzles, and is interested in the underpinnings of medicine, you should explore what we do at the FDA. We often have openings, and they're posted on USAjobs.gov. We look for people who understand data analysis and research or are interested in learning, and who have a public health outlook.

BIOSTATISTICIAN

Job Description

Biostatisticians use statistical expertise to help researchers investigate issues in all areas of public health. There are biostatisticians at the FDA who develop mathematical models to help find the best ways to do clinical trials. Biostatisticians review data sent in by drug manufacturers to see if their study results match the claims they are making. Some create mathematical models to predict how drugs will be processed by the body or use statistical techniques to help determine if a generic drug is equivalent to the brand-name version. Biostatisticians also analyze data to check the quality of drugs and other medical products.

Typical tasks for a biostatistician might include figuring out how many patients are needed for a clinical trial, determining how many measurements should be taken, and calculating whether a result is likely to represent a real effect or is probably due to chance. If a study isn't done correctly the information may be useless, so biostatisticians help look for pitfalls in how data will be gathered and errors in study design. Biostatisticians are involved in many different areas of public health, in addition to drug safety. This is primarily a desk job, with a lot of computer time. Biostatisticians often work with a team of other public health experts, such as epidemiologists, medical officers, research scientists, and policy analysts.

Education and Certification

Biostatisticians have training in mathematics and statistics, as well as knowledge of how medical research is done. For some jobs, a bachelor's degree in mathematics or statistics will suffice, but a master's or doctoral degree allows for far more opportunities. Jobs in research and in academia usually require a PhD.

Core Competencies and Skills

- Knack for numbers
- Strong understanding of statistics
- Basic understanding of epidemiology
- Excellent computer skills, particularly with statistics programs
- Willingness to continue learning (statistical methods are constantly evolving)
- Ability to "translate" statistical information into language that nonstatisticians can understand.
- Understanding of how to apply statistical and mathematical concepts to real-world situations

Compensation

For all statisticians, the median salary in 2008 was $72,610, and most earned between $40,000 and $117,000. According to a survey by the American Statistical Association (ASA), government statisticians with master's degrees or PhDs earn about $60,000 to $150,000, with salaries increasing with experience and responsibility, and PhDs earning somewhat more than those at the master's degree level. The salary range in a recent ASA survey of academic institutions was similar.

Workplaces

Biostatisticians are employed in virtually every aspect of public health. Within the federal government, those who focus on drug safety work largely at the FDA, but there are many biostatisticians at CDC, NIH, and other agencies within HHS. Biostatisticians also work for health departments, nonprofit organizations, medical centers and hospitals, and consulting firms.

Employment Outlook

Biostatisticians are needed for a wide range of research, safety, and health surveillance projects. In recent years, there has been a shortage of biostatisticians with training at the graduate level, so there should be very good opportunities for employment.

For Further Information

- American Statistical Association (ASA)
  www.amstat.org
- American Public Health Association—Statistics Section
  www.apha.org/membergroups/sections/aphasections/stats

DIRECTOR, STATE BOARD OF PHARMACY

Job Description

A state board of pharmacy is the regulatory agency for the practice of pharmacy in that state. The board is usually responsible for licensing pharmacies and pharmacists; regulating drug storage, security, and dispensing; and inspecting pharmacies, drug distributors, and manufacturers. The pharmacy board also handles complaints and imposes penalties when people and businesses violate regulations. It informs pharmacists of changes in laws and regulations and provides guidance regarding the scope of what pharmacists can do.

Overseeing all the board's work is the executive director, who advises the members on policy matters and strategic planning, guides the implementation of policies, and supervises certain staff members. The executive director must be aware of pharmacy issues and trends, current laws and policies, pending legislation, and issues in inspection, licensing, and enforcement. Day-to-day tasks can include attending legislative hearings, working on ways to improve processes for licensing or inspection, addressing budget issues, and collaborating with other agencies.

Education and Certification

Some states, but not all, require the executive director to be a licensed pharmacist, and many require a certain amount of experience. Knowledge of pharmacy laws and regulations and of how the board of pharmacy functions is essential. Some executive directors have come to the job after serving as appointed members.

Core Competencies and Skills

- Strong managerial skills
- Excellent negotiating and public speaking skills
- Ability to handle multiple responsibilities at once
- Interest in policymaking
- Talent for networking and making connections with legislators, government officials, and local leaders in the pharmacy world
- Thorough understanding of pharmacy laws and regulations
- Ability to communicate complex information to people from many different backgrounds

Compensation

Salaries vary substantially by state, ranging from about $80,000 to $125,000.

Workplaces

State boards of pharmacy may be separate agencies or may be located within health departments, departments of consumer affairs or public safety, departments of regulation and licensing, or other sections of state government. In some states, the director of the board of pharmacy also oversees other agencies, as well.

Employment Outlook

Each state has only one pharmacy board, and these jobs are generally filled by people who have experience with the activities of a state pharmacy board.

For Further Information

■ National Association of Boards of Pharmacy (NABP)
www.nabp.net
■ National Association of State Controlled Substance Authorities (NASCSA)
www.nascsa.org

REGULATORY AFFAIRS SPECIALIST

Job Description

A regulatory affairs specialist is in charge of making sure that a drug company is complying with legal and regulatory requirements. Regulations come into play at all steps of the process from research to marketing, including conducting clinical trials, applying for the FDA approval (or approval from agencies in other countries), and manufacturing the drug. A regulatory affairs specialist ensures that an application for a new drug contains all the necessary documents and information. During the research stages, a regulatory affairs specialist examines plans for clinical trials, ensures they conform to requirements, and keeps track of what forms must be submitted and what information must be reported. There are also regulatory affairs specialists involved in drug advertising and promotion. Responsibilities include reviewing advertising copy and label information to be sure they contain essential information and don't make any claims that aren't allowed.

Education and Certification

Most regulatory affairs specialists have at least a bachelor's degree, and a major in a scientific or health-related field is helpful. Many have completed at least some graduate work or hold higher degrees. There are now some degree and certificate programs specifically in regulatory affairs, but it is not yet clear how important this type of background will be. Experience in research, laboratory work, clinical medicine, pharmacy, or a related area is often expected, and experience with the FDA is helpful. Experience with project management can also be useful. Some jobs require specialized knowledge, such as an engineering background for work related to medical devices. Companies may also look for employees with certain certifications. Regulatory affairs specialists may be more competitive if they hold Regulatory Affairs Certification from the Regulatory Affairs Professionals Society.

Core Competencies and Skills

- Patience with paperwork
- Ability to understand complex technical and legal language
- Strong sense of ethics
- Basic understanding of science, medicine, and research principles
- Familiarity with applicable federal requirements
- Good computer skills, including word processing and spreadsheets
- Ability to keep important company information confidential

Compensation

A salary in the range $50,000 to $60,000 is not unusual for a lower-level job. An experienced regulatory affairs specialist can earn a salary in the $100,000 range.

Workplaces

Regulatory affairs specialists involved in health care work primarily for industry, and sometimes for medical centers, universities, research companies, or other organizations that must meet certain requirements.

Employment Outlook

Because pharmaceutical and medical device companies can't run without making sure they comply with regulations, these jobs will likely be secure. In recent years, companies have had difficulty finding qualified people to do this work, but they are often looking for seasoned professionals. One way to get started is to begin with a company in a different role and look for opportunities to learn about regulatory affairs.

For Further Information

- Regulatory Affairs Professionals Society (RAPS)
  www.raps.org

9

Environmental Health and Water Safety

The environment has always had an impact on public health practice, since the earliest development of city water supplies and sewage systems. In modern times, however, public health and environmental health have become somewhat separated. The 1988 report from the Institute of Medicine, *The Future of Public Health*, pointed out that this fragmentation impeded coordination of health efforts and led to inadequate attention to the connection between environmental problems and health.

In recent years, public health experts have begun to pay increasing attention to possible links between environmental hazards and disease. In fact, the CDC is now planning an environmental public health tracking network. Researchers are studying the effects of air pollution and chemical exposures through food, water, and personal care products. The impact of the built environment is a current hot topic: Can our neighborhoods make us sicker or healthier? Does a lack of sidewalks contribute to obesity? There is much we don't know about environmental health. Many chemicals used in industry have unknown potential health impacts. Issues such as the health consequences of climate change, environmental radiation exposures, and other pollutants are all subjects of study. As we learn more, there may be increasing opportunities to contribute to public health by focusing on our interaction with the environment.

There is a great deal of information at the CDC's National Center for Environmental Health (www.cdc.gov/nceh) and their consumer information site on environmental health (www.cdc.gov/Environmental). The National Institute for Environmental Health Sciences (www.niehs. nih.gov) is another good resource. APHA has a section dedicated to environmental health and a special Web site at www.ephs-apha.org.

Job opportunities in environmental health are broad. In addition to this chapter, see also the entries for epidemiologist, medical epidemiologist, public health nurse, biostatistician, injury prevention specialist, poison information specialist, health educator, health promotion coordinator, disease ecologist, and study coordinator, and the chapter on Occupational Health.

TOXICOLOGIST

Job Description

In public health, toxicologists study the effects of drugs, poisons, environmental contaminants, and other potentially dangerous substances, and then they use that knowledge to help protect the public's health and safety. Some specialize in certain substances or certain aspects of health, such as cancer risk or effects on the nervous system. Others focus on certain locations, such as factories where chemicals are produced or used. Often, it is not simply the presence of a substance that is important, but the amount, the way it is used, and potential interactions with other substances. In addition to environmental health issues, there are toxicologists working in other areas of public health such as helping figure out if a medicine, a food preservative, or an ingredient in lipstick poses any risk. Toxicologists who focus on research might do laboratory work, or they might help figure out if a chemical is causing an outbreak of illness. Toxicologists are also involved in creating and enforcing regulations to ensure that industries produce, use, and dispose of chemicals safely. They often must be able to explain the science behind their recommendations to nonexperts, such as legislators, health department personnel, and company workers.

Education and Certification

About half of all toxicologists have PhDs. Bachelor's and master's degree training are also options, but people with doctoral degrees will likely have the best opportunities. Many toxicologists start with an undergraduate degree in a science such as chemistry or biology, then go on to more specialized graduate study. Physicians, veterinarians, and people with PhDs in other biomedical sciences can pursue postdoctoral training in toxicology. Several certifications are available. The American Board of Toxicology recognizes expertise in general toxicology, and the American Board of Applied Toxicology focuses specifically on the study of poisons as they affect humans and animals. Both organizations require a PhD or a combination of education and experience. The American Board of Emergency Medicine certifies physicians with a subspecialty in toxicology.

Core Competencies and Skills

- Knack for biology, chemistry, math, and statistics
- Ability to learn complex new information rapidly
- Interest in scientific detective work
- Good writing and speaking skills to communicate your findings or explain risks and regulations
- Understanding of research design and implementation
- At least basic knowledge of epidemiology and biostatistics
- Knowledge of biochemistry, molecular biology, and physiology
- Knowledge of known toxins and their effects on the body
- For work in industry and government, especially, the skills to interact effectively with a team

Compensation

Toxicologists can earn quite a good living, depending on level of education and type of employer. A new PhD graduate might earn between $35,000 and $60,000, with compensation rising to $70,000 to $100,000 with a decade of experience. Industry tends to offer higher salaries than academic institutions, and a PhD will generally earn more than someone with less education. Toxicologists who become corporate executives can earn quite a bit more.

Workplaces

About 15% of toxicologists work for city, state, and federal government institutions. About 20% are employed by universities, where their jobs can include both doing research and teaching students. About half work for private employers such as manufacturers and pharmaceutical companies. Toxicologists are also found at nonprofit organizations and consulting firms.

Employment Outlook

The job outlook for toxicologists is good. There is a strong need for the kind of work toxicologists do, and the specialized training helps reduce competition from other types of scientists.

For Further Information

- Society of Toxicology (SOT)
  www.toxicology.org
- American College of Toxicology (ACT)
  www.actox.org
- American Academy of Clinical Toxicology (AACT)
  www.clintox.org
- American College of Medical Toxicology (ACMT)
  www.acmt.net

POISONING PREVENTION COORDINATOR

Job Description

The coordinator of a poisoning prevention program manages outreach, education, and clean-up programs to remove dangerous substances from the environment. Many poisoning prevention programs are focused on reducing the risk of lead poisoning in children. Depending on the program, the coordinator's tasks might include maintaining a registry of houses and apartments without lead contamination, directing people to professionals who can help with lead removal, and organizing a program to screen children for elevated lead levels. The coordinator is often responsible for managing employees and takes part in handling the budget, including writing grant proposals and administering grants. Obtaining and analyzing local data is another typical task. The coordinator may be directly involved in activities such as conducting community outreach and educational sessions, providing counseling to families when children have elevated lead levels, inspecting homes, and training housing contractors, or they may delegate such tasks to staff members. He may also help to develop new programs, based on available funding and local needs. The job can include policy and advocacy work, as well. Often, it involves meeting with partner organizations to share ideas and encourage cooperation.

Education and Certification

Poisoning prevention coordinators are often nurses or trained health educators. A bachelor's degree and experience overseeing a community service or health-related program will meet some employers' requirements. An MPH can be helpful, and a master's degree in either public health or a related field is sometimes required. Certification as a lead inspector, which requires a short course and an examination, may be needed if inspection is part of the job.

Core Competencies and Skills

- Excellent organizational and managerial skills
- Ability to multitask
- Flexibility to work with many different types of people, from community members to city leaders
- Strong writing and spoken communication skills
- Knowledge of public health program administration and the ability to interpret regulations
- Working knowledge of epidemiology, data analysis, and program evaluation techniques
- Ability to create educational programs and materials geared to the needs of local communities
- Knowledge of issues specific to the prevention program, such as lead poisoning risks and abatement requirements

Compensation

Salaries vary widely. Examples include the low $20,000s at a small non-profit, about $40,000 with a larger organization, and mid $50,000s or $60,000s at various health departments.

Workplaces

Poisoning prevention programs are located in city, county, and state health departments, and there are also programs run by nonprofit organizations and academic institutions. Although jobs will be different than those in local communities, there is also work in lead poisoning prevention at the federal level: The CDC has a lead prevention program, which works with local programs as well as providing information for health care providers and the public, and there are lead prevention efforts at the EPA and at the Department of Housing and Urban Development.

Employment Outlook

There are many childhood lead poisoning prevention programs throughout the United States, at state and local health departments. When a city or county health department has its own lead prevention program, it will usually have only one or two coordinator positions. However, there are other opportunities to be involved in these programs and to gain experience. In addition, there are other programs focusing on the prevention of poisoning through environmental exposures, including pesticide poisoning and exposure to lead in the workplace.

For Further Information

■ CDC Lead Poisoning Prevention Program
www.cdc.gov/nceh/lead

ENVIRONMENTAL ENGINEER

Job Description

Environmental engineers (also called sanitary engineers) who work in public health are involved in fields such as air pollution control, waste disposal, and water treatment. They may design systems to keep drinking water supplies safe, to control pollution, to treat wastewater and sewage, and to manage potentially hazardous waste. They may help track down problems at existing facilities, and develop regulations to guide future efforts. When a developer is building a new subdivision, it is an environmental engineer who looks over the plans for the proposed water supply. These engineers also ensure that projects comply with laws and regulations. They need not only to understand the principles of design and development but also to have at least basic knowledge of pathogens, disease vectors, toxicology, and other public health issues.

Other typical jobs include working on systems to treat wastewater from manufacturing plants, finding ways to reduce emissions from automobiles or factory smokestacks, planning for the safe disposal of dangerous substances, and finding ways to clean up contaminated sites. In the course of their work, environmental engineers interact with other experts, including health officials, architects, and building contractors. They are often based primarily in offices, but they typically spend about a quarter of their time on-site, inspecting locations or facilities. There are also environmental engineers who primarily do research on environmental control.

Education and Certification

Environmental engineers need at least a bachelor's degree in a related engineering field, and a master's degree in environmental engineering can lead to better employment opportunities; academic programs should be accredited by the Accreditation Board for Engineering and Technology. A PhD is not essential for most environmental engineers but can open up additional possibilities, especially for those interested in research. Engineers who plan to offer their services to public or private clients need to hold a state license and to be certified as Professional Engineers (PE). Engineers who work for government agencies often need a license and PE certification, and certification is generally necessary for advancement.

Core Competencies and Skills

- Tendency to be detail-oriented and analytical
- Strong skills in math and physics
- Curiosity about science and biology
- Understanding of the workings of state or local government, including how government policies can affect engineering projects
- Ability to communicate with scientists and nonscientists in different fields
- High-level computer skills, for the use of technical design and modeling programs and data analysis
- Ability to visualize projects, such as imagining two-dimensional plans in three dimensions

Compensation

In 2008, the median salary for an environmental engineer was $74,000. The top 10% earned more than $115,000, and only 10% earned $45,000 or less. More experience and more education will generally lead to higher compensation. The federal government and private industry tend to pay more than state governments, although salaries vary.

Workplaces

Environmental engineers work for city, county, and state governments, usually either with the health department or with a separate division focused on the environment. They also work for corporations that contract to do government work. Some work directly for a corporation in a specific industry.

Employment Outlook

Overall, opportunities for engineers should be in rough balance with the number of people looking for jobs. The prospects for environmental engineers are expected to be particularly good. With increasing attention to the nation's infrastructure, a growing population, and an increasing emphasis on preventing environmental problems and hazards, the need for engineers with expertise in water supply and pollution control is likely to increase.

For Further Information

- American Society of Civil Engineers (ASCE)
  www.asce.org
- American Academy of Environmental Engineers (AAEE)
  www.aaee.net
- American Waterworks Association (AWWA)
  www.awwa.org

PUBLIC HEALTH PROFILE: Environmental Engineer
Jeff Stone, PE
Chief Engineer
Engineering Section, Arkansas Department of Health, Little Rock, AK

Describe the sort of work you do.

We protect the public's health with regard to drinking water and wastewater as well as ensure compliance with the federal Safe Drinking Water Act. We approve or disapprove water sources, drinking water treatment plant designs, wastewater treatment plant designs, and treated wastewater discharge locations. We monitor everything from the source to the wastewater plant and back to the river.

Continued

I manage a staff of engineers and engineering technicians. The technicians carry most of the on-site inspection burden and also review the data from drinking water treatment plants each month. The district engineers carry most of the burden of plan review, both for new sites and for infrastructure improvement, and they do some of the inspections of larger systems and sources.

What is a typical day like at your job?

My door is always open to my staff. People come to confirm judgment calls or to obtain guidance. There are also calls from outside consultants and design engineers. They might call to get my input before they get started on projects. When an issue in the field warrants my first-hand experience, I'll go out. If there's a breakdown of equipment or a treatment interruption that could lead to contamination, we swing into action and try to prevent disease from happening. The health agency has an emergency office manned 24/7. If there's a power failure that makes our water utilities not operational, or if there's a water main break, I get a call.

What education or training do you have? Is it typical for your job?

I have a bachelor's in chemical engineering and an MBA, and I am licensed as a PE. Some people in this field have a bachelor's degree in civil or chemical engineering and a master's degree in environmental engineering. That master's would give them a bit of an edge. But many environmental engineers don't actually have a degree in "environmental engineering." Their degree is in, say, civil engineering and their work experience and acquired competency is in environmental engineering.

What path did you take to get to the job you are in today?

I started out working in industry, but the technical skills I was learning were specific to that business. I wanted a skill set that would lead me through a forty or fifty year career, and I decided on environmental engineering. I found an ad in the newspaper for a job at the health

Continued

department. I had taken some electives in environmental engineering at college, and that may have helped me get the job. After I started here, I became licensed as a PE, and I advanced to jobs with more responsibility. I earned the MBA for my own interest and to learn about finance, personnel law, and other things that a manager needs to understand.

Where might you go from here, if you wanted to advance your career?

I think I have a lot of choices. I've been here with the health agency about 24 years and worked my way up. If I stayed here I might have a chance at higher positions, or I could start a second career after I retire and become a project manager with a consulting engineering company.

What is the worst or most challenging part of your job?

Even though my department is trying to help the public, we still have to deal with people who are upset by things that have happened. Also, my decisions can mean a cost difference to utilities in building their systems, or they can affect someone's property rights. If someone thinks my decision is incorrect or unfair, they can appeal my decision or perhaps litigate. I've never been subpoenaed for a court case, but I've had to answer difficult calls. This is not a job for people who can't deal with conflict in a calm way and strive to find solutions to problems.

What is the best part?

I'm involved in important judgment calls and in responding to emergency situations, and I know that what I do matters. The general public might not be aware of exactly what my department does, or of the problems we prevent, but they rely on us to keep them safe.

What advice do you have for someone who is interested in your career?

Anyone, in any kind of engineering, should pursue professional licensure. Not only does it enhance your own marketability, it is also the best way I know of to have a career that serves you over your lifetime.

HAZARDOUS WASTE INSPECTOR

Job Description

The job title isn't glamorous, but hazardous waste inspectors have very important jobs. They ensure that manufacturers meet local and national guidelines for the disposal of certain types of potentially dangerous waste. They keep our water supply safe and keep dangerous substances out of our soil and air. They visit factories and other industrial settings to help companies understand and comply with waste management regulations. Some serve as site assessors, taking soil samples at vacant properties to determine if hazardous substances are present. They also inspect waste treatment and disposal facilities, and they respond to complaints about improper dumping or disposal. Inspections may require travel throughout the state, including nights away from home. Back at the office, inspectors write reports, research current regulations, interact with other inspectors, and talk with industry managers or clients.

Education and Certification

A typical requirement is a bachelor's degree in environmental science or a related field, or college-level science classes plus related training. Some jobs require specific certification. Courses and certificates are available at some colleges and universities and from professional organizations.

Core Competencies and Skills

- Basic grounding in chemistry, biology, and geology
- Interest in educating workers as well as in uncovering problems
- Strong organizational skills and self-motivation
- Ability to write technical reports
- Understanding of local and national waste disposal and management regulations
- Interest in work that involves travel to multiple sites as well as office work

Compensation

State health department salaries vary according to local budgets as well as cost of living and level of responsibility. Some examples include

$40,000 to the low $50,000s in one northern state, $44,000 to $60,000 in a southwestern state, and up to the $80,000s on the west coast.

Workplaces

State governments employ hazardous waste inspectors, usually through the state environmental agency, to inspect businesses throughout the state. There are also some opportunities for hazardous materials inspectors in city and county programs. Manufacturers employ people with similar knowledge to oversee waste management within their companies. Industrial waste disposal companies also employ inspectors to make sure they are transporting materials safely and complying with the law.

Employment Outlook

Government jobs are considered relatively stable, even in tough economic times, and in fact some supervisors report that it can be challenging to find qualified employees for this type of work.

For Further Information

- Environmental Council of the States (ECOS)
  www.ecos.org
- Environmental Protection Agency—Wastes Web site
  www.epa.gov/wastes

PUBLIC HEALTH PROFILE: Hazardous Waste Inspector
Chad Babcock
Environmental Project Scientist
South Dakota Department of Environment and Natural Resources, Pierre, SD

Describe the sort of work you do.

I work in the waste management program of South Dakota's Department of Environment and Natural Resources. My primary job involves inspecting commercial businesses and government agencies for compliance with hazardous waste rules and inspecting facilities

Continued

permitted to accept solid waste for treatment, storage, or disposal. During hazardous waste inspections, I ensure that businesses and agencies properly determine if wastes they generate are ignitable, corrosive, or toxic, and I make sure the wastes are managed accordingly.

What is a typical day like at your job?

Some days I'm out of the office doing inspections, and other days I'm here completing inspection reports and preparing for upcoming inspections. I plan a series of inspections once or twice a month. To prepare for each inspection, I go through all our records on the company, and I put together a preinspection report. I'll look for any compliance issues in the past. Then I call the company to schedule my visit. When I go do the inspection, I like to start by sitting down with a company representative to get an idea of what the company does and the waste that they generate. Then I get out into the actual manufacturing or production area. I walk through, discuss each process, and inspect waste storage areas. If I identify anything new or unexpected, I'll request additional information. I usually have a number of questions to follow up with afterward, so after I return to the office I'll contact the company representative again as needed. Finally, I write the official report.

Sometimes I handle complaint calls and do complaint investigations. This usually involves contacting affected parties to gather information about the incident. Many times I will conduct a follow-up inspection. People will also call with questions about the hazardous waste rules that apply to them, or if they have a new manufacturing process they might ask for our assistance.

What education or training do you have? Is it typical for your job?

I have a bachelor's degree in biological chemistry, with a minor in math and physics. A bachelor's degree in life or physical sciences or in an engineering discipline is pretty typical for this job.

What path did you take to get to the job you are in today?

I started out working as a research scientist with an animal vaccines company. I was working mostly in a laboratory. I had more of an interest in environmental health than I did in the animal work, so when I

Continued

moved to a new city, I began working as an environmental consultant. I think my science background helped me get that position. I did a lot of asbestos and lead paint inspections for renovation and demolition work, also some on-site monitoring. I kept an eye out for openings in the Department of Environment and Natural Resources, and when I saw one advertised, I applied.

Where might you go from here, if you wanted to advance your career?

Experience is valued a lot here, and there are always opportunities to take on new tasks without changing levels. Right now I'm not that interested in supervising. I am more interested in increased responsibilities involved in inspecting, permitting, and compliance assistance. I report to a senior scientist who manages the hazardous waste program and an engineering director who manages the solid waste program.

What is the worst or most challenging part of your job?

Tracking the disposal of different wastes involves a lot of paperwork, and that gets tedious at times. Report writing involves evaluation, which I find interesting, but also has some aspects that are repetitive.

What is the best part?

I really enjoy the background research for inspections and reports. There is a lot of learning and often unique application of regulations, so it remains challenging and interesting. And then, I like taking that knowledge and discussing company operations with personnel of various levels. There is constantly something different and I have the opportunity to meet and work with an interesting group of people.

What advice do you have for someone who is interested in your career?

It is helpful to have a background in chemistry, biology, and environmental science. I value my experience as a consultant, working with businesses and seeing how they do things, because it gave me a good perspective on both sides of what I do now. I think it helped me understand my current job a lot more quickly, coming from the background that I had.

HYDROLOGIST

Job Description

Hydrologists study the occurrence, movement, and distribution of water on and within the earth, and the relationship between that water and the surrounding environment. Hydrologists also look at how water can become contaminated or purified by natural processes, and they develop methods to predict changes and monitor effects. Hydrologists who work with public health officials are involved in monitoring water supplies, looking for pollutants, and determining how altering certain aspects of the environment could influence water purity. If a new well is planned, a hydrologist will look at how it could affect water in existing wells. They also help decide where to place new waste disposal facilities, to minimize environmental effects. The job often includes work in the field, as well as high-tech work such as statistical modeling and the use of remote sensing technologies. Hydrologists work closely with engineers, geologists, and other experts.

Education and Certification

A master's degree is standard. There are some entry-level jobs for people with bachelor's degrees, and high-level research jobs tend to require PhDs. Degrees specifically in hydrology are available, but many programs have a hydrology concentration within a degree program in geoscience, engineering, or environmental science. There are also nondegree certificates available from some universities, for people who already have a background in a related subject. Several states require hydrologists to be licensed if they will be offering their services to the public. There is also a voluntary certification available from the American Institute of Hydrology (AIH).

Core Competencies and Skills

- Good math and statistics skills and an interest in the natural sciences
- Strong computer skills, for statistical and modeling programs
- Ability to collaborate with other scientists
- Ability to communicate information to nonscientists
- Training in how to assess risk and apply theory to actual practice
- Understanding of public health laws and regulations as they relate to environmental issues

- Knowledge of geology, chemistry, physics, and biology with respect to water systems
- Knowledge of how various water contaminants can affect human health

Compensation

In 2008, the median salary for hydrologists was about $71,000. The top 10% earned more than $105,000 and the bottom 10%, about $44,000 or less.

Workplaces

There are many different types of jobs, with varying levels of connection with traditional public health issues. About 27% of hydrologists work for the federal government, primarily with the U.S. Geological Survey and the Department of Defense, although not all are directly concerned with public health issues. At state environmental agencies, hydrologists work with engineers and others concerned with the supply and safety of our water and with waste management. There are also many jobs for hydrologists at consulting firms and in industry, and there are opportunities at nonprofit organizations concerned with the environment.

Employment Outlook

Opportunities for hydrologists should be good. Changes in government regulations are expected to create new jobs. Population increases, with ongoing development of environmentally sensitive areas, as well as climate change will likely increase the need for hydrologists, as well.

For Further Information

- American Institute of Hydrology (AIH)
  www.aihydrology.org

ENVIRONMENTAL HEALTH NURSE

Job Description

Environmental health nursing could be considered a subset of public health nursing. These nurses focus on specific dangers in the environment, from lead exposures to air pollution. To help control asthma in a community, a nurse might learn about all the environmental triggers—such as dust mites, pet dander, and other indoor pollutants—and then help develop programs and policies to reduce exposures at home and school. An environmental health nurse may work with other environmental health experts, health care providers, community groups, and even builders and contractors. Often, the job involves going out into the community—including homes, schools, and hospitals—to assess potential dangers and offer interventions. There can also be a lot of deskwork, including data collection, analysis, and writing.

Education and Certification

The best preparation is a master's degree in environmental health nursing. There are only a few such programs now, but more will probably be offered in the future. Other options include a master's in occupational health nursing, which covers many environmental health hazards, or an MPH in addition to a nursing degree.

Core Competencies and Skills

- Interest in community-level health
- Desire to work collaboratively across health disciplines
- Interest in health care policy
- Ability to understand not only environmental risk factors but the social factors that contribute to those risks
- Knowledge of epidemiologic principles and techniques
- Training in how to design and carry out public health programs
- Knowledge of toxicology and environmental health risks

Compensation

The specific responsibilities of environmental health nurses can vary widely, so it is difficult to give a typical salary. For nurses in general, typical salaries range from about $40,000 to $90,000.

Workplaces

Environmental health nurses work for local and state health departments, but also for hospitals, schools, and industry—both at factories and in office settings. There are also opportunities in federal government, including the CDC and EPA.

Employment Outlook

Environmental health nursing is an emerging field. Many health departments have lead abatement programs, and the federal government has been putting increasing amounts of funding into grants for environmental health nursing research and programs. The job outlook is still uncertain but likely to be favorable as more is learned about the connection between environment and health.

For Further Information

- Alliance of Nurses for Healthy Environments (ANHE)
  www.e-commons.org/anhe
- Agency for Toxic Substances and Disease Registry (ATSDR)
  Environmental Health Nursing Initiative
  www.atsdr.cdc.gov/EHN

COMMUNITY ACTIVIST

Job Description

Community activists are involved in many aspects of public health, including environmental health. These committed workers take on issues that are important to the health of a group, a neighborhood, or a city as a whole, and they help community members make their voices heard. Sometimes, a campaign begins with a single individual who rallies others to the cause; sometimes, it is the result of a concern that many people share. Either way, a community activist's work involves bringing people together (through meetings, events, and online forums) to find ways to solve problems. They encourage interest through news stories, local events, and social marketing campaigns. They work with legislators and public officials when possible, but when necessary they use legal challenges, protests, and staged events to make their voices heard. Members of community-focused organizations might be found collecting signatures for a petition to stop the city from building a bus depot near a school. They may meet with local business leaders to get funding to build a park. They might attend a hearing about new regulations to reduce pollution in a local river. Or you may spot them at a playground, taking soil samples to test for lead. Often, community action organizations are small, so just a few people share many responsibilities, including raising funds, writing press releases, planning events, and speaking to the public. When these organizations have more employees, jobs are more clearly delineated; see the section on jobs at nonprofit organizations for more details.

Education and Certification

A community activist can have any educational background, from a high school diploma to a doctoral degree. There is no special certification. People with specific degrees may be able to put them to use in their work. For example, someone with a degree in environmental science might be able to speak with particular authority about pollution, and a nurse might use her knowledge to explain health effects to legislators or the public.

Core Competencies and Skills

- Excellent interpersonal skills
- Dedication
- Ability to see a project through to completion
- Resilience to deal with disappointments and setbacks
- Strong writing skills for creating grant proposals, press releases, and other documents
- Good research skills, to learn about the issues and about the science and medical facts involved
- Knack for seeing all sides of an issue and understanding how different people think
- Belief that it is possible to change the status quo

Compensation

People who work for community activist organizations do their jobs for the opportunity to make a difference. Salaries depend greatly on the specific job description and on the organization's funding but are often less than someone with the same skills and education would earn in the private sector. At a small grassroots organization, an entry-level salary in the $20,000 to $30,000 range would not be unusual for someone with a bachelor's degree; a larger organization, or one in an area with a high cost of living, might start even entry-level workers at $35,000 or more. Typical salaries for jobs requiring a master's degree or more experience can start in the mid $30,000s to mid $40,000, again with higher compensation in certain situations. The director can expect to earn more, for example $60,000 at a small organization or $75,000 at a midsized one.

Salaries also vary according to the organization's structure, and a group may choose to pay more to recruit and retain the most qualified people.

Workplaces

Community activists work for nonprofit organizations, often small or medium-sized organizations that focus on a specific region or issue. There are also large, national nonprofits with divisions devoted to grassroots work, but the issues being addressed will generally be less specific to the local community. If there is an important local issue that is not being addressed, starting an organization is also an option. It is a risk, and it takes a great deal of commitment, but if it succeeds it can make a real difference to the community.

Employment Outlook

There is always work to be done to help make our communities healthier, but the local organizations that do this work often have limited funding so it may take a while to find a job in a specific area of interest. One way to get started is to volunteer, get to know people involved in the cause, and let it be known that you're interested if a job opens up.

For Further Information

- Idealist
  www.idealist.org

PUBLIC HEALTH PROFILE: Community Activist
Peggy Shepard
Executive Director
WE ACT for Environmental Justice, New York, NY

Describe the sort of work you do.

WE ACT is a nonprofit organization. We work to build community power among people of color in northern Manhattan neighborhoods, in order to improve environmental health, environmental protection, and policy. We do that through research, training of community members, mobilization of the community, and working in public policy.

Continued

We got started in the late 1980s, after a new sewage treatment plant began spewing noxious odors and fumes that were making people sick. We convinced the city to spend millions of dollars to fix the plant. Today, we have many different projects and programs. We have been educating people in our local community about climate change, and we are also doing policy work on the city and state level. On the national level, we recently held the first climate justice conference in the country. Some of our other concerns include clean air and water, indoor air quality, sanitation, transportation, and the development and use of our waterfront.

What is a typical day like at your job?

I can give you a better idea by looking at a week. Last week, on Monday I gave a talk about food security and food justice at a large meeting put together by the City Council president. Then I had a paper due for an upcoming conference. On Tuesday I had a meeting with our board about fundraising, a meeting with one of my staff about performance planning, and a call with a consultant about the theory of change. I had a conference call with the CDC for their National Conversation on Chemicals and Public Health. I lead a workgroup called Serving Communities. That night, I had a board meeting with the Public Health Association of New York City.

Wednesday, I had a meeting with a major media organization to talk about diversity issues, and I had a meeting at the Environmental Defense Fund, where I co-chair the environmental justice committee. That was a brainstorming session to talk about new directions. Then, I had a call with the Children's Environmental Health Network to discuss their climate change policy initiative. Later in the week I had a fundraiser with a Harlem community group, and I had a meeting with the founding dean of a new School of Public Health, to brainstorm about a new initiative to work on heath disparities in Harlem.

What education or training do you have? Is it typical for your job?

I have a bachelor's degree in English and background in journalism. Mostly, what you need is commitment. Business skills are helpful, too. WE ACT is a nonprofit, but all the things you have to do with a small business, you have to do with a nonprofit as well.

Continued

What path did you take to get to the job you are in today?

I had worked for 10 years as a journalist, a magazine editor, a speech-writer, and a public information director for a state agency. I used my writing skills to work in political campaigns, and I became the public relations director for Jesse Jackson's first campaign for president. After that, I ran for the office of Democratic District Leader for West Harlem. When I was elected, the community asked me to help them organize to address the problems with the sewage plant.

Then, we found out that the Metropolitan Transportation Authority (MTA) was building another bus depot in our community. Diesel exhaust contributes to multiple health problems. We already had multiple bus depots in northern Manhattan, whereas other communities had none. We decided to file a lawsuit against the MTA—and to do that, your group needs a name, and official members. We began developing WE ACT officially, so we were able to file that lawsuit. The city settled our lawsuit for $1.1 million, and it was decided that WE ACT would get $200,000 to staff the organization. That's when I started my job as director.

Where might you go from here, if you wanted to advance your career?

I could probably have a position at the EPA or at the state Department of Environmental Conservation. A lot of government agencies don't know very much about how to interact with community, so I have a lot to offer. Or, I could move into community-based research. But right now I'm where I want to be.

What is the worst or most challenging part of your job?

Funders will support programs and projects, but they don't usually want to give general operating money. We know what it takes to make a really strong, viable organization, but we don't always have the money to hire the additional staff that would make everyone's job here easier.

What is the best part?

The best part is taking community concerns and developing solutions that are realized. To give you a case in point—we had a dilapidated

Continued

waterfront. We organized the community to envision a waterfront park, and we got the city to build it! It is also very gratifying to help support the development of a national voice on environmental justice.

What advice do you have for someone who is interested in your career?

You have to be at the right point in your life cycle, and you also have to have the right family situation. Your family has to be extremely supportive. You'll be giving 200% every day for a long time.

HEALTH PHYSICIST

Job Description

Health physics focuses on making it possible for radiation to be used for beneficial purposes. Health physicists are experts in radiation safety, and they work at many different levels and in a variety of settings to protect workers, the public, and the environment. One role is in the licensing and inspection of radioactive materials, which are used in many different industries. Health physicists also observe the workers in these settings, ensure they are taking appropriate precautions, and offer training and guidance when needed. They judge whether safety measures are acceptable.

Health physicists are also involved in planning for radiation safety. Some help design facilities with proper radiation control and create training programs for employees. There are health physicists at nuclear power plants, ensuring compliance with regulations, training workers, and monitoring safety measures. Some health physicists work primarily in emergency preparedness, such as modeling the potential effects of a radioactive dispersal device (a "dirty bomb") and teaching first responders how to deal with a radiation emergency. There are health physicists figuring out how to decontaminate sites where military facilities, research laboratories, or industrial operations used to be. There are also opportunities for these experts in research, in policy and regulations, and in many other areas of health-related work.

Education and Certification

An associate's degree can suffice for certain jobs such as inspecting x-ray equipment, but most jobs in health physics require a minimum of a bachelor's degree in a field such as physics, engineering, or environmental health. It is possible to earn a bachelor's, master's, or PhD degree specifically in health physics, although not all universities offer these degrees. Health physicists also need specific training in radiation safety and preparedness, which is usually obtained on the job. Experience is enough to allow career advancement in some settings, and there is a wide range of interesting jobs for which a master's degree is sufficient. Some high-level jobs require a PhD. Voluntary certification as a Certified Health Physicist (CHP) is available through the American Board of Health Physics.

Core Competencies and Skills

- Knack for math and physics and at least basic knowledge of biology and chemistry
- Strong sense of responsibility and ethics
- Good writing and organizational skills
- Ability to interpret situations and make appropriate decisions with limited guidance
- Ability to gather information and apply it to real-world situations
- For inspectors, especially, willingness to travel
- Knowledge of local and federal regulations pertaining to radiation
- Knowledge of radiation hazards, safety measures, and monitoring

Compensation

According to a 2009 CHP salary survey, the median salary for a CHP is about $116,000 per year, but this likely reflects a certain subset of workers. Top salaries tend to be in industry and at nuclear power plants. Salaries for state inspectors can be substantially lower, in the range of around $60,000.

Workplaces

Health physicists can be found wherever radiation is involved. There are inspectors at state health departments, and a few large metropolitan areas have local programs. There are many opportunities in the federal government, including at the Nuclear Regulatory Commission (NRC) and the CDC. There are health physicists working in research laboratories, at decommissioning facilities, and in industry. Some health physicists teach and do research at universities. There are also "medical health physicists" who focus on radiation safety and radiation therapy at medical facilities.

Employment Outlook

There is currently a shortage of health physicists, and future opportunities for employment look promising. Actual opportunities will depend on the setting and the number of qualified job applicants. There seems to be more awareness of jobs in medical physics (e.g., at hospitals and medical centers), suggesting that there may be less competition for health physics jobs; some state supervisors note that it can be difficult to find a qualified applicant, while others have noted an uptick in qualified candidates. There are often jobs available at the federal level for people with appropriate experience and training. With more nuclear power plants expected to be built over the next few decades, there will likely be an increased demand for health physicists to train employees and oversee safety.

For Further Information

- Health Physics Society (HPS)
  www.hps.org
- American Nuclear Society (ANS)
  www.ans.org

REFERENCE

Institute of Medicine Committee for the Study of the Future of Public Health. *The future of public health*. Washington, DC: National Academies Press, 1988.

10 Occupational Health and Safety

The health of our workers has an enormous impact on the health of our population as a whole. With 3.7 million nonfatal work-related injuries and illnesses and about 5,000 deaths in 2008, there are many opportunities to improve health and safety on the job. Occupational health and safety experts approach a given industry's or company's workers not just as individuals but as a population facing certain risks and hazards. They use the techniques of public health to address health and safety concerns and reduce risks in the workplace. In fact, the training for occupational medicine physicians incorporates earning an MPH.

There are two federal agencies concerned with occupational health. The National Institute for Occupational Safety and Health (NIOSH) is an agency within the CDC (www.cdc.gov/niosh). Over at the Department of Labor, the Occupational Safety and Health Administration (OSHA) develops, implements, and enforces workplace standards for occupational safety and health (www.osha.gov). There are also state health departments that do their own surveillance and interventions. Many government agencies employ occupational health experts to protect their workers' health, and there are extensive opportunities in the private sector.

In addition to the careers discussed in this chapter, there are many other professionals working in this field, including epidemiologists, toxicologists, environmental health nurses, and health promotion program coordinators.

OCCUPATIONAL MEDICINE PHYSICIAN

Job Description

Occupational medicine is a medical specialty that has a lot of overlap with public health. "Occ med" physicians are trained to look at the health of workers as a population, as well as to know about all the different medical issues that can arise in the workplace. Office workers can suffer injuries from repetitive tasks or even badly made chairs. Warehouse workers can hurt their backs. Factory workers can be exposed to heavy metals, dust, dangerous equipment, and loud noise. The occupational medicine physician watches for these types of injuries and sounds the alarm if a pattern or serious danger exists. For example, if several factory employees develop breathing problems, the physician might investigate the cause. An outbreak of the flu can tear through a company; the occupational medicine physician helps devise and promote ways to prevent such outbreaks.

In their day-to-day work, these physicians treat injured or ill workers, make official determinations about whether injuries and illnesses are work related, and help workers get back on the job. When workers develop physical or mental illnesses that do not have occupational causes, they help guide them to outside care and make recommendations for any needed work accommodations. Occupational medicine doctors also work with other experts to help companies put safety measures into place, like muting loud sounds that can damage hearing.

Education and Certification

An occupational medicine doctor needs an MD or DO and a current license to practice. The doctor must also have completed a residency program in occupational or occupational and environmental medicine. Board certification, which involves passing a rigorous examination after finishing residency, is not absolutely essential, but it is often expected. It is also possible for physicians in other medical specialties to acquire skills in occupational medicine through continuing education and on-the-job training.

Core Competencies and Skills

- Familiarity with the industry or industries in which the patient population works

- Good interpersonal skills
- Curiosity and a willingness to investigate when the source of an illness is not clear
- Knowledge of medicine, in general, and of hazards present in the workplace
- Knowledge of rehabilitation methods for injured workers
- Knowledge of workplace safety and sanitation issues
- Knowledge of workers' compensation laws and of local, state, and national regulations that apply to worker safety and health

Compensation

The starting salary for an occupational medicine physician is often at or above $100,000 per year. According to the American College of Occupational and Environmental Medicine (ACOEM), in 2006 the median salary for someone board certified in occupational medicine was $175,000.

Workplaces

Some occupational medicine physicians work directly for large companies. Others work with practices focused on occupational medicine or with groups of doctors from various specialties. These doctors see patients who are employed by many different companies and have work-related complaints. The practice of occupational medicine often includes both direct patient care and visits to worksites. There are also jobs in government, consulting, and academia.

Employment Outlook

The outlook for employment should be good; the demand for occupational medicine physicians is estimated to be greater than the supply of physicians trained in this specialty.

For Further Information

- American College of Occupational and Environmental Medicine (ACOEM)
  www.acoem.org
- American College of Preventive Medicine (ACPM)
  www.acpm.org

EMPLOYEE HEALTH NURSE

Job Description

A nurse who works in employee health is responsible for certifying employees are physically fit and assisting with the care of workers who have been injured; he or she also does work that helps keep a whole population of workers healthy. Like an occupational medicine physician, the employee health nurse must be alert for outbreaks of illness and patterns of injury that could signal a safety problem. He or she encourages employees to have annual flu shots and practice good hand hygiene. If the workplace is a health care center, employees must be tested routinely for tuberculosis and have other immunizations verified, so that they do not expose patients to dangerous diseases. The employee health nurse conducts any required drug tests. When workers are injured, the employee health nurse may be the one to manage and coordinate their care. Responsibilities may also include counseling workers with substance abuse problems or psychosocial concerns. Many employee health nurses are involved in writing health-related newsletters, teaching employees about safety and infection control, designing health-promotion programs, and making decisions about safety in the workplace.

Education and Certification

Employee health nurses are usually RNs, and some are nurse practitioners. They must be licensed in the state where they practice, and a bachelor's degree is helpful. Also helpful is certification as a Certified Occupational Health Nurse by the American Board of Occupational Health Nurses. Some jobs also ask for other certifications related to the work, such as Certified Health Education Specialist. Precise job requirements vary according to the setting and workers' needs. Nurses who want to further their careers and obtain upper-level positions helping to shape occupational health programs or policy, for example, at government agencies or in industry, can benefit from earning an MPH with a focus on occupational health, a combined MSN/MPH, or even a PhD.

Core Competencies and Skills

- Familiarity with medical billing and coding
- Excellent communication skills

- Understanding of the company culture
- Background in worksite wellness or general health promotion
- Knowledge of workplace safety and health issues, OSHA regulations, and workers' compensation laws
- Ability to apply research findings and recommendations to real-life needs
- Knowledge of how to interpret data on workers' health
- Skills to design, implement, and evaluate health and safety programs that will have an impact on workers

Compensation

The median salary for an RN in 2008 was about $62,000 per year, with most earning between $43,000 and $92,000. According to a 2006 report from the American Association of Occupational Health Nurses (AAOHN), the average salary for members was $63,472, with higher education and certification associated with higher salaries.

Workplaces

Employee health nurses work for hospitals, factories, railroads, retail businesses, and universities—essentially, any type of company, organization, or agency with enough workers to justify having a department dedicated to their health. Nurses in the broader category of occupational health also work for private medical practices, government agencies, and research universities.

Employment Outlook

The demand for nurses is expected to be high over the next several years. Opportunities for occupational health nurses will likely be good, as companies recognize the value of systematically protecting and promoting workers' health.

For Further Information

- American Association of Occupational Health Nurses (AAOHN) *www.aaohn.org*

INDUSTRIAL HYGIENIST

Job Description

The field of industrial hygiene involves the anticipation, recognition, evaluation, and control of occupational health hazards. Industrial hygienists examine workplaces for potential health and safety hazards and make recommendations about what should be done to improve the safety of the workers. This includes not only recognizing current hazards but anticipating future ones. "Workplaces" can be dangerous places like factories and mines, but they can also be academic settings, hospitals, and corporate offices. Industrial hygienists deal with many different types of hazards—noise that can damage hearing, chemicals that can irritate skin, fumes that can damage lungs, and more. They also work to prevent repetitive stress injuries and physical damage due to other causes. They look for ways to reduce the chance that workers will be exposed to a hazard in the first place. They limit risk further through policies that encourage safe work habits. When necessary, they recommend personal safety measures, such as masks and earplugs; if workers are not following the recommendations, they determine why not and how to increase compliance. Industrial hygienists can also be involved in scientific research. Some participate in determining national regulations and standards. Some do disaster preparedness work, such as helping local EMS professionals understand what chemicals are used at a worksite.

Education and Certification

An industrial hygienist has at least a bachelor's degree in a field such as physics, chemistry, biology, or engineering. Many choose to pursue a master's degree focusing on industrial hygiene, an MPH with an emphasis in industrial hygiene, or a master's in a related field. The exact expectations and requirements vary according to the job. A Certified Industrial Hygienist credential is available for industrial hygienists who have met academic requirements, have several years of experience, and pass a certifying examination. Although certification is not required, employers do tend to prefer it.

Core Competencies and Skills

- Good attention to detail
- Knack for the physical sciences

- Appreciation for technical work and measurement
- Good observational skills
- Ability to communicate clearly with employees from entry level to administration
- Good memory for rules and regulations, combined with knowledge of local and federal requirements for the workplace
- Willingness to get dirty during inspections at worksites or on factory floors

Compensation

The median salary for all occupational health and safety specialists, a category that includes industrial hygienists, is about $62,000 per year. A starting salary for someone just out of school might be as low as $35,000 to $40,000, but someone with the Certified Industrial Hygienist credential can expect compensation closer to the $60,000 to $70,000 range. With experience and increasing responsibility, salaries can rise to $90,000 or more.

Workplaces

Industrial hygienists work in many different industries, wherever workers' safety is a concern. They also work at federal government agencies such as OSHA and NIOSH. Many industrial hygienists travel to worksite locations to do inspections and observe practices, which can require them to face the same (potentially dangerous) conditions that onsite workers do. Others spend much of their time in an office setting.

Employment Outlook

The demand for people who work in occupational health and safety is expected to expand from 2006 to 2016, due to advances in technology and changes in regulations. The health of the economy will influence the need for industrial hygienists, because demand depends on the expansion of businesses. Government jobs tend to be more stable.

For Further Information

- American Industrial Hygiene Association (AIHA)
  www.aiha.org
- American Conference of Governmental Industrial Hygienists (ACGIH)
  www.acgih.org

- APHA section for Occupational Health and Safety
www.apha.org/membergroups/sections/aphasections/occupational
- American Society of Safety Engineers (ASSE)
www.asse.org

PUBLIC HEALTH PROFILE: Industrial Hygienist
Erica Stewart, CIH, HEM

National Environmental, Health and Safety Senior Manager
Kaiser Permanente, Oakland, CA

Describe the sort of work you do.

I work for Kaiser Permanente, the oldest and largest not-for-profit health care organization in the country. In addition to direct patient care settings, we have laboratories, steam plants, distribution warehouses, and optical lens production facilities; we even do construction. My job involves creating standards and policies that will prevent exposures to hazardous substances, or to conditions that could be dangerous. I also collaborate with different departments to come up with solutions to occupational health problems. Kaiser Permanente is very supportive of outside volunteer activity, and so I've been able to become involved in a NIOSH initiative called Prevention by Design. We're looking at preventing occupational injuries from occuring by designing the workplace to anticipate and mitigate hazards.

What is a typical day like at your job?

My typical day consists of answering emails, meeting with people, and working on projects. One project I'm working on is creating hazardous materials inventories for new hospital construction. That means making lists of what materials will be found in each department and in what quantity, and then creating tables that compare the maximum allowable amount to the amount needed. The lists include all kinds of hazardous substances—even hand sanitizer. I'm also working with our National Facilities Services group, the department that sets our building standards.

I do four or five audits a year, where I go out to see what our employees actually do in practice versus what the policy says they should do, or what they say they are doing. The audits take about 60 hours, with

Continued

3 days on the site plus preparing and writing the report. I do department tours, interview employees, assess metrics, and calculate scores.

What education or training do you have? Is it typical for your job?

I have a bachelor's degree in biochemistry, and I'm a certified industrial hygienist. I'm also a certified health care environmental manager. It's common for people at my level to have graduate degrees, usually a master's in industrial hygiene or occupational and environmental health and safety.

What path did you take to get to the job you are in today?

My stepfather was an industrial hygienist, and he suggested that I go to work in an industrial hygiene lab. I thought it was really cool. You get to see what people do and then help make the work easier on them. I started doing different kinds of fieldwork, like testing emissions from manufacturing plants, and lab work like spectrophotometry. Later, I did asbestos abatement project management, directing the safety aspects of the work. My first job at Kaiser Permanente was as an Industrial Hygiene Technician, doing air sampling in sterile processing, in the lab, and in the operating room. I've been here for 19 years now, with progressive levels of responsibility.

Where might you go from here, if you wanted to advance your career?

The next step might be Director or Senior Director, or even Vice President, but I'm satisfied with where my career is now. I enjoy doing work that demands technical expertise, as well as managing people, and a higher-level title might mean that I'd be doing more managing and less technical work. I like to keep that balance of sharp technical skills while still mentoring and coaching junior staff.

What is the worst or most challenging part of your job?

Working with different kinds of people can be challenging. Sometimes it takes all of my skills to make sure I'm working on the problem and not the personality. It's not a matter of whether we like each other,

Continued

but whether the problem is solved. You have to look at it from their perspective, so you get cooperation rather than resistance.

What is the best part?

My favorite thing is coming up with solutions to problems that have seemed intractable. It's really rewarding when I'm working with a group of people and we come up with something that is quantifiably better than it was before, and everyone benefits.

What advice do you have for someone who is interested in your career?

I don't think there's any one path to getting involved in this career. It can be through education and training, or doing fieldwork, or doing research. You can work in manufacturing, consulting, or services such as health care. I happen to like dealing with engineering controls, while other people are more interested in doing training or air sampling. You do bring the experience from each job to your next one, so you can change from one focus to another. For those who are looking for advice I would also say find your local professional organization and get involved. Local chapters of AIHA are very helpful for networking.

CORPORATE MEDICAL DIRECTOR

Job Description

Physicians who serve as corporate medical directors can be in charge of many different aspects of health within a company. The exact responsibilities vary according to the size, type, and values of the corporation. At a large company, the corporate medical director's job can encompass worksites from offices to factories, at locations around the country or around the world. The medical director often oversees employee health services, deciding what will be offered at on-site medical clinics and ensuring that protocols are in place to address illnesses and on-the-job injuries. He may oversee preventive care programs—such as serving healthier food in the cafeteria or rewarding employees for getting fit. He may also advise on workplace hazards, such as identifying toxic substances and safety issues in the workplace. He may be in charge of protecting the health of employees who have to travel overseas, ensuring that they know where to get essential vaccinations and have somewhere to turn if they get sick while away. He guides the preparations for emergencies and disease outbreaks at company worksites. Some medical directors are primarily administrators, while others also provide patient care. Some are involved in health-related research pertaining to company products and in monitoring consumer complaints about injuries or illnesses. This job usually has regular business hours, although there may be after-hours calls for emergencies, and physicians generally use their own time to keep up with medical journals and research news.

Education and Certification

A corporate medical director needs an MD or DO degree and a current license to practice. For those who provide direct patient care in multiple locations, licensure in more than one state may be needed. Typical specialties are internal medicine, family medicine, or occupational medicine; training in occupational medicine or in preventive medicine and public health is particularly useful and can be an advantage when seeking a job.

Core Competencies and Skills

- Strong communication skills, including both writing and public speaking
- Good managerial skills
- Understanding of how the business world works
- Knowledge of epidemiology and the ability to interpret data
- Awareness of issues that arise in medical practice on the population level, in addition to one-on-one patient care
- Good understanding of occupational health issues, particularly regarding the work that the company does or products it manufactures
- Ability to work with business executives who may not understand the principles of occupational medicine and public health, and to educate them as necessary

Compensation

Physicians who share their expertise as corporate medical directors can expect to be well paid. At smaller companies, they may work as part-time contractors, earning from $100 to $300 per hour depending on their experience and skills, as well as on the local market. Typical salaries range from the mid to high $100,000s, for example, at a large manufacturing plant, to well over $200,000 for a high-level director at a major corporation. According to ACOEM, in 2006 the median salary for a corporate medical director was $193,000.

Workplaces

Corporate medical directors work at all sorts of companies, from manufacturing to office settings.

Employment Outlook

Most large companies offer some type of employee health services, although not all will have their own, extensive health programs. For that past few years, there has been a lot of talk about employee health promotion as a way to keep insurance costs down and productivity up, so there may be expanding opportunities. Typically a corporate medical director needs some experience in occupational settings and administrative work; one way to obtain this experience is to start by working part-time with smaller companies or as an occupational medicine physician in one division or location.

For Further Information

■ See the organizations listed with occupational medicine physician.
■ American College of Physician Executives
  www.acpe.org

PUBLIC HEALTH PROFILE: Corporate Medical Director
Ron Stout, MD, MPH
Medical Director
Procter & Gamble, Cincinnati, OH

Describe the sort of work you do.

I've been at Procter & Gamble for 10 years and served as medical director across a number of different units. Right now, I'm in the

Continued

Health & Wellbeing Global Business Unit. That includes prescription drugs, over-the-counter medications, oral care products like toothpaste, feminine hygiene products, pet care, and snacks. I have three different roles—employee health, safety surveillance for our products, and medical affairs.

In employee health, my responsibilities include monitoring, maintaining, and improving the health of employees across the world. We do a lot of traditional occupational health, but in the last several years we have really recognized that general health and productivity go hand in hand. So we're very focused on prevention. For product safety surveillance, I make sure that we respond to customer concerns, and I review aggregate data to see if there are any problems with our products. Medical affairs includes everything from engaging thought leaders to help us develop new products, to serving as principal investigator on research studies. I'm also involved in some wonderful partnerships. We've partnered with the CDC to develop a product that purifies water for drinking at a cost of less than a penny for 10 L, and we've been working on combating the arsenic contamination of wells in Bangladesh.

What is a typical day like at your job?

I usually start at 6:30 or 7 a.m. to handle international calls and emails. Then from about 7:30 to 9 a.m., we have leadership meetings. Sometimes it's the global physicians, or the business unit physicians, or people on a development project. Then I'll have project-specific items throughout the day. If we're launching a new product, I'll review the active ingredients and see if there are safety issues in manufacturing. I'll collaborate with our industrial hygienists to develop surveillance protocols or techniques for handling ingredients safely.

When I'm in charge of a study, I meet with the project team to understand the objective and help design the research. I keep up with the literature on preventive medicine and primary care, and on illnesses that our products treat. Another common task is handling human resources issues. I'm in charge of emergency response, too. We're trying to have automated external defibrillators available within 4 minutes for every employee around the world, so I might have a meeting with a vendor about how to do that. I'm also one of the people who gets called if a hurricane or flood affects one of our plants.

Continued

What education or training do you have? Is it typical for your job?

I have an MD and an MPH. I'm board certified in public health and general preventive medicine, occupational health and environmental medicine, and family practice. I've studied epidemiology, and I've done a lot of industry-specific trainings. Other corporate medical directors have different combinations of training and experience, so it's hard to say exactly what would be typical.

What path did you take to get to the job you are in today?

Since my family didn't have the money to put me through college, I enlisted in the Air Force. They paid for college and medical school, and then I had a service requirement. I did some clinical work, but mostly I did program planning and leadership. After I came out of active duty, I became the medical director for preventive medicine and occupational services at a medical center. I came to Procter & Gamble after that.

Where might you go from here, if you wanted to advance your career?

I've had the opportunity to run a department in a government agency, so that would be one possible place to go from a job at this level. I've also thought about running for Congress. I could go back to clinical practice, I could return to a small company where I'm the only medical person around, or I could go work directly for a non-governmental organization and learn more about implementing the public health and development plans we develop.

What is the worst or most challenging part of your job?

It's a challenge to constantly have to work in a consensus-driven environment. We move people around often within the company—so if there was consensus yesterday, there might not be today.

What is the best part?

My favorite part is the work we do to improve health in the developing world and to provide disaster relief when it is needed. I'm

Continued

helping to leverage a wonderful company's assets to directly make a difference.

What advice do you have for someone who is interested in your career?

Once you've determined your passions, recognize that you must be a life-long learner. It's not so important who educates you, but to whom you remain connected. Your educational journey will give you relationships that will benefit you throughout your career. Look for experiences that will give you connections to the thought leaders, the innovators, the people on the cutting edge. Look for mentors, it makes all the difference.

REFERENCES

Bureau of Labor Statistics. *Economic news release: Census of fatal occupational injuries summary, 2008*. August 20, 2009. http://www.bls.gov/news.release/cfoi.nr0.htm accessed March 23, 2010

Bureau of Labor Statistics. *Economic news release: Workplace injuries and illnesses—2008*. October 29, 2009. http://www.bls.gov/news.release/osh.nr0.htm accessed March 23, 2010

11 Food Safety and Nutrition

When Upton Sinclair wrote *The Jungle*, he was hoping to raise awareness about abuses suffered by the American working class. But his book—detailing disgusting practices in the Chicago meatpacking industry—had an entirely different effect. An official report on the meatpacking industry confirmed much of what Sinclair had written. In 1906, Congress passed the Federal Meat Inspection Act, mandating certain inspections and sanitary standards.

1906 was also the year Congress passed the Food and Drugs Act, which laid out certain requirements for food. In the years since then, food safety regulations and requirements have been strengthened and expanded. Today, thousands of researchers, inspectors, educators, administrators, and others keep an eye on the food supply from farm to table and work to ensure that imported food is safe to eat.

Just because our food is very safe, though, doesn't mean we're always eating right, as the epidemic of obesity demonstrates. Both inadequate nutrition and obesity-related diseases are important problems which concern many public health professionals.

Two good places to begin learning more about food safety and nutrition are the FDA and USDA Web sites (fda.gov and usda.gov) and the Web site nutrition.gov.

The careers described in this chapter are just an introduction to the many jobs concerned with the foods we eat. Others include health teacher, health educator, health promotion coordinator, WIC nutritionist, community health worker, deputy director/family health services, and study coordinator.

NUTRITION CONSULTANT

Job Description

Public health agencies and nonprofit organizations have many different programs to promote good nutrition. There are federal nutrition assistance programs like WIC, the School Breakfast Program, the Administration on Aging Nutrition Program, and the Child and Adult Food Care Program. There are also initiatives to encourage healthful eating and to combat obesity. These include improvements in the quality of school lunches, efforts to increase access to healthful foods, and even gardening, cooking and nutrition classes.

Public health nutrition consultants contribute to these programs in many different ways. A consultant may work on developing the policies and standards that guide local or national efforts. He or she may provide technical assistance at the state or local level, training staff members as they develop their own programs or implement state or national initiatives. The consultant can help when program leaders are not particularly knowledgeable about the nuances of nutrition. He or she may assess statewide or local needs and evaluate programs, gathering and analyzing data to see if they are making a difference in levels of obesity, consumption of healthy foods, or other goals. Some consultants participate in community outreach directly, while some coordinate the work of community health workers, nutritionists, or other staff. The job can include collaborating with other agencies and local organizations. A consultant may also prepare reports and presentations to share with legislators, the media, and the general public.

Education and Certification

Nutritionists need to have at least a bachelor's degree with a focus on nutrition, or a bachelor's plus additional nutrition-related coursework. Often, although not always, jobs for nutrition consultants require the registered dietitian credential from the Commission on Dietetic Registration at the American Dietetic Association. At least a year or two of relevant experience is usually expected, and a master's degree in nutrition, an MPH, or a master's degree in a related subject can make a candidate more competitive. A graduate degree also increases opportunities for upper-level positions. A nutritionist may need a license to practice, depending on the state.

Core Competencies and Skills

- Interest in the connection between food and health
- Sensitivity to diverse cultures, with the ability to adjust recommendations to cultural preferences and needs
- Up-to-date knowledge about the connections between nutrition and health
- At least basic knowledge of statistics and epidemiology, with the ability to interpret local and national data and study results
- Ability to develop programs appropriate to a given population's needs
- Knowledge of laws and regulations regarding public health nutrition programs
- Excellent verbal and written communication skills and a knack for teaching

Compensation

In 2008, the median salary for dietitians and nutritionists was about $51,000. Only 10% earned less than $31,000, and 10% earned more than $73,000.

Workplaces

Actual job titles vary, but nutritionists doing these types of work are found at public health agencies and programs from the city to the federal level. Examples of employers include "healthy city" initiatives, state health departments, WIC and other USDA-sponsored programs, and the CDC. There are opportunities at nonprofit organizations that focus on nutrition and disease prevention, in employee health and wellness programs, in programs at medical centers, and with consulting firms. Jobs with titles such as "nutrition program manager" and "nutrition program coordinator" often incorporate similar responsibilities.

Employment Outlook

Nutritionists with graduate degrees will likely have the best opportunities. Concerns about obesity and the diabetes epidemic have led to an increasing emphasis on the role of diet in disease prevention; assuming funding is available, this may lead to a greater role for nutritionists in public health.

For Further Information

■ Association of State and Territorial Public Health Nutrition Directors (ASTPHND)
www.astphnd.org
■ Also see the organizations listed under WIC Nutritionist.

FOOD SERVICE SANITARIAN

Job Description

A sanitarian applies environmental control measures to protect human health and safety. (Sanitarian is an old term; today's sanitarians are often called "environmental health specialists.") Food service sanitarians are experts in the food safety issues that arise in places where food is prepared and served. Many work as city or county health inspectors. They visit restaurants, grocery stores, and other food sales outlets, as well as places like school cafeterias, daycare centers, and nursing homes, to see whether they are in compliance with city and state food safety codes. They look at how food is stored, cooked, handled, and transported. They ensure the premises are clean, they check for vermin, and they observe the workers. If they find something wrong, they issue citations and make recommendations about how to correct the problem. Sanitarians also investigate calls from consumers about food poisoning or about practices that look unhygienic. Another role for these inspectors is to review food safety plans submitted by restaurants before they open. If the location of the sinks, for example, looks likely to lead to problems, the sanitarian can offer constructive advice. In some areas, the food service inspector also has other environmental health responsibilities, such as inspecting swimming pools or investigating stream pollution and other community hygiene violations.

Education and Certification

Requirements for food service sanitarians vary. Many health departments require a bachelor's degree including substantial study of the biological and/or physical sciences, but some will accept an associate's degree with appropriate experience in food safety or environmental health. Some states require an examination and special licensing or registration. In addition to state credentials, the National Environmental Health Association offers a Registered Environmental Health Specialist/ Registered Sanitarian certification; candidates must have either a bachelor's degree in environmental health or a degree in a different subject plus certain coursework and experience.

Core Competencies and Skills

- Attention to detail
- Knowledge of food safety
- Willingness to inspect places that may be dirty or unpleasant
- Strong sense of ethics, including the willingness to stand behind the inspection results even if a restaurant owner or worker at an inspected facility objects
- The ability to offer constructive criticism and education
- Familiarity with regulations regarding food service and environmental health

Compensation

Typical salaries for environmental health specialists range from about $40,000 to $70,000 per year.

Workplaces

Food service sanitarians often work for health departments and other government agencies. They are also employed in the private sector, such as for restaurant chains, where they do quality assurance and risk management work.

Employment Outlook

Health inspector jobs tend to be fairly stable, because state regulations create an ongoing need. Overall, there is likely to be demand for sanitarians as interest in food safety and other environmental health issues increases.

For Further Information

- National Environmental Health Association (NEHA)
  www.neha.org
- National Association of County and City Health Officials—
  Environmental Health
  www.naccho.org/topics/environmental

PUBLIC HEALTH PROFILE: Food Service Sanitarian
Sara T. Losh, RS
Health Inspector
Health and Food Safety, City of Frisco, Frisco, TX

Describe the sort of work you do.

My department is responsible for inspecting all retail food establishments in Frisco, TX. That includes restaurants, convenience stores, schools, and daycare centers. Each place is inspected from one to four times a year depending on its risk category, which is determined by the type of food and population they serve. When a new retail establishment is being built, we review the plans, and then we do a courtesy walk-through to make sure they are on the right track. We do a final health inspection before they can open.

What is a typical day like at your job?

Most days I start in the office, although some days I may start with inspections in the field. When I'm doing an inspection, I enter the establishment and ask for the person in charge. I ask to see their health permit and certified food manager's certificate. Sometimes the owner or manager accompanies me on the inspection, sometimes not. I begin by washing my hands, and I'll check for hot water at the same time. Then I start in the back, looking at the kitchen and storage areas, and work around to the front. I look for insects and rodents, check food temperatures both on the line and in coolers, and check expiration dates. I also make sure the food comes from an

Continued

approved source; for example, it can't be something that was made at home and brought in. I look for hair restraints on employees and make sure workers are not touching ready-to-eat foods with their bare hands. I look to see that floors, walls, and ceilings are in good repair and that drains are working properly.

Most places pass their inspections. Occasionally an establishment does have to be closed for an imminent health hazard. I have the manager lock the door and post a sign that they are temporarily closed, and as customers leave the door is locked again behind them. We try to keep closings to a limited time, because we don't want restaurants to lose business, but they have to pass inspection to be able to open again.

What education or training do you have? Is it typical for your job?

I have a bachelor's in nutrition with a minor in business administration, which from my experience isn't typical at all. Registered sanitarians tend to have degrees in environmental health or one of the hard sciences.

What path did you take to get to the job you are in today?

I learned about this field in college. I was studying nutrition, and I actually overheard someone having a conversation about the type of work I'm doing now. I got a job supervising food service at a hospital and assisting the dietitian, but at the same time I studied on my own for the state RS examination. When I passed that, I answered an ad in the paper for a health inspector job with the city of Dallas. I came to work for the city of Frisco a few years later because it was an easier commute. I heard about the job through the Texas Environmental Association, which usually announces openings at their quarterly meetings.

Where might you go from here, if you wanted to advance your career?

I would accept a promotion if a position became available, but I am happy where I am right now. The next level from here would be a senior health inspector or supervisor position.

Continued

What is the worst or most challenging part of your job?

I don't like writing citations and fining people. Depending on how an establishment works, sometimes the manager has to pay the fine even if the problem is not his fault. Sometimes people get fired because of citations. I'm just doing my job, but I don't enjoy that part.

What is the best part?

It is especially satisfying to be able to catch something that might have made someone sick. People can die from foodborne illness, and I can help prevent that. Also, sometimes people in the establishments really don't know the right thing to do, and I can educate them.

What advice do you have for someone who is interested in your career?

When I started as an RS, I had never worked in the food industry before, and I had a lot to learn about that. My suggestion is to get into food service and do that for a while, so you know what it is like to be on the other side. I think people with that experience pick up things faster. They know how the dish machine works, and they know how the service industry works. If you are in a food service job, look at the health inspector's report and talk to the inspector when he or she comes in. They will be more than happy to talk with you.

FOOD INSPECTOR/DEPARTMENT OF AGRICULTURE

Job Description

Food inspectors at the USDA or state agricultural departments verify the safety of meat, poultry, dairy products, and eggs, and of products made from these foods. They're involved in every step of food production, from commercial slaughterhouses and dairy farms to the assembling of TV dinners or the making of ice cream. Most inspectors at the USDA's Food Safety and Inspection Service start in privately owned slaughter plants, where they examine animals both before and after slaughter. At processing plants, inspectors help assure the safe production of foods made with animal products. An import inspector is stationed at a port or border crossing and is responsible for examining food that is being brought into the country.

Inspectors who want to advance their careers can seek promotion to more complex or less physically strenuous jobs. One career path at the USDA is to the position of consumer safety inspector. Consumer safety inspectors are assigned to one or more plants, where they make sure that sanitation standards are being met and that plans for food safety are properly formulated and carried out. Their responsibilities include working with plant managers, owners, and workers to explain regulations and address any violations; conducting samplings and surveys to assess potential problems; and making sure that products are accurately labeled.

Education and Certification

Food inspectors at the USDA need either a bachelor's degree, including a certain number of hours studying the biological, physical, mathematical, or agricultural sciences, or experience that pertains to what an inspector needs to know. They must also pass a written test. Consumer safety inspectors need either experience as an inspector (or in a similar position), or a bachelor's degree with a substantial amount of relevant coursework such as agricultural, biological or physical science, food technology, nutrition, engineering, or epidemiology.

Core Competencies and Skills

- Attention to detail
- Honesty, with the ability to stand by a decision
- Interest in the science of food safety
- A strong stomach
- Willingness to handle animal carcasses and to be in an environment where animal-based food products are made
- Ability to handle relatively strenuous work
- Knowledge of laws and regulations regarding food safety

Compensation

For agricultural inspectors in general (not just food inspectors), the median salary in 2008 was about $41,000 per year, with most earning between $25,000 and $59,000. The USDA food inspector salaries range from about $30,000 to $50,000.

Workplaces

Many inspectors work for the Food Safety and Inspection Service at the USDA. State departments of agriculture also hire inspectors to inspect slaughter plants, dairy farms, and processing plants. Private companies hire inspectors to make sure they are complying with regulations. There are also inspectors involved in fruit and vegetable production.

Employment Outlook

The U.S. Department of Labor estimates that over the next several years, job openings for agricultural inspectors will be in rough balance with the number of people seeking jobs. As of 2009, the USDA was actively seeking qualified applicants to fill food inspector jobs and offering bonuses for those willing to work in certain locations.

For Further Information

- United States Department of Agriculture Food Safety and Inspection Service (FSIS)
  www.fsis.usda.gov
- National Association of State Departments of Agriculture (NASDA)
  www.nasda.org

CONSUMER SAFETY OFFICER/FDA

Job Description

Consumer safety officers (CSOs) at the FDA fill many different roles related to the public's health and safety; food safety is one of the areas in which they work. Depending on the specific job, a CSO involved in food safety might be assigned to inspect factories where food products are made, warehouses where food is stored, or companies that handle distribution. CSOs make recommendations when violations are found and prepare written reports. When inspections lead to administrative hearings or judicial proceedings, they may be called to testify. They may also investigate complaints about food-related illnesses or about manufacturers' production processes. CSOs can work their way up to higher-level positions. There are CSOs who serve as consultants and advisors, who help shape policy, and who manage projects and programs. They may evaluate state programs to be sure they adhere to national guidelines, advise industry on the interpretation of regulations, assess new technologies to determine whether regulations should be changed, and train other CSOs. Some CSOs serve as division directors, overseeing multiple staff members and taking on significant administrative and leadership responsibilities.

CSOs are located both at the FDA headquarters in Washington, DC, and throughout the United States, and some jobs involve significant travel. The job can have standard working hours, or—for certain inspectors, for example—it may include regularly scheduled weekend work.

Education and Certification

CSOs can qualify for entry-level jobs either through education or a combination of education and experience. The minimum education requirement is a bachelor's degree with significant study of the biological sciences, physical sciences, nutrition, or other fields related to the work. Alternatively, a CSO can have some college-level work (30 semester hours of relevant study) plus experience or other education that meets the needs of the job. Higher-level positions require further education or additional relevant experience.

Core Competencies and Skills

- Attention to detail
- Ability to make independent judgments
- Interest in food manufacturing and safety
- Understanding of how to assess safety risks
- Ability to understand complex regulations and apply them to real-world settings
- Good communication skills, including writing skills

Compensation

The FDA CSOs who serve as inspectors in the food industry typically earn about $26,000 to $62,000 per year. Those who advance to supervisory positions or to positions requiring work of significant complexity and responsibility can earn substantially more, with salaries eventually reaching $100,000 and above.

Workplaces

The FDA employs a large number of CSOs. The Office of Regulatory Affairs is the primary department concerned with compliance and enforcement, with investigators who inspect the whole range of FDA-regulated products. There are also CSOs in other FDA centers, including the Center for Drug Evaluation and Research, the Center for Biologics Evaluation and Research, the Center for Devices and Radiological Health, and the Department of Regulatory Affairs.

Employment Outlook

CSO is among the jobs included in a current FDA hiring initiative, so opportunities should be good. As of 2010, the FDA Web site featured a list of job fairs and professional meetings that recruiters would be attending.

For Further Information

■ FDA Office of Regulatory Affairs (ORA)
   www.fda.gov/AboutFDA/CentersOffices/ORA

FOOD SCIENTIST

Job Description

A food scientist is just that—a scientist who studies food. It is a broad field, ranging from nutrition to safety. Many food scientists work in industry, helping to develop new products, but they play an important role in public health, too. There are researchers studying food safety, including how much pesticide is found in food, or whether genetically modified plants are safe. When a manufacturer proposes a new technology for pasteurizing or preserving food, food scientists test and evaluate the method to be certain it is effective. Some food scientists study food packaging to evaluate how long a product will stay fresh and how to reduce the risk of contamination. Others look at how well preservatives work or how bacterial contamination spreads. There are jobs related to toxicology, exploring the potential effects of specific foods, preservatives, or packaging on people's health. Another focus is nutrition, such as studying the effect of cooking or canning on nutritional content or finding ways to add vitamins without changing the taste. There are food scientists involved in cutting-edge research, as well. All of this is primarily laboratory work.

On the regulatory side, food scientists help develop and implement new regulations and standards for keeping food safe. They gather information from the laboratory scientists and write recommendations, often combining deskwork with visits to factories and laboratories. Some food scientists inspect manufacturing facilities, and some provide education to the public or to manufacturers. Some are involved in protecting the international food supply. Some focus on risk analysis and its application to practice and policy.

Education and Certification

A bachelor's degree in food science will suffice for some jobs, but salaries are lower and the level of responsibility is generally less than with a graduate degree. A master's degree opens up more opportunities and allows for more specialized work. Many people who do food science research at the FDA have PhDs, but there are also opportunities for people with a bachelor's or master's degree. Some food scientists choose to earn MPH degrees, in addition to their other education, to broaden their knowledge of public health issues.

Core Competencies and Skills

- Curiosity and creativity
- Strong critical thinking and reasoning ability
- Good mathematical skills
- Understanding of how and why people make choices about what they eat
- Respect for food as a biological material
- Patience and the ability to see projects through to completion
- Knowledge of food production processes, quality control issues, and other elements of preparing and packaging food for sale
- Understanding of biology and chemistry as it relates to food

Compensation

A survey of members of the Institute of Food Technologists found that in 2009, the average salary for a beginning food scientist with a bachelor's degree was about $50,000; with a master's, about $61,000; and with a PhD, $75,000. The median salary for all members was $87,700, and people with extensive experience were earning over $100,000 per year. In 2008, the U.S. Department of Labor estimated that the average salary for all food scientists and technologists was around $60,000, with most earning between $34,000 and $105,000 per year.

Workplaces

In the federal government, food scientists work primarily for the FDA and the USDA. There are jobs at state health departments and departments of agriculture, as well, depending on local needs and budgets. There are opportunities with nonprofit organizations, trade associations, and with individual companies. Some food scientists with doctoral degrees are researchers or professors at universities.

Employment Outlook

Schools that train food scientists say that most students have secured jobs before graduation. The employment outlook for food scientists is expected to remain good, especially for those with master's degrees. Increasing interest from the federal government and the public on food safety and nutrition could also lead to new opportunities.

For Further Information

- Institute of Food Technologists (IFT)
  www.ift.org
- International Association for Food Protection (IAFP)
  www.foodprotection.org
- American Institute of Chemical Engineers (AIChE)
  www.aiche.org

REFERENCES

Sinclair, U. (1906). *The Jungle*. Project Gutenberg EBook, released March 11, 2006. Retrieved from http://www.gutenberg.org/etext/140

Swann, J. P. (1998). *FDA's origin and functions*. Retrieved from http://www.fda.gov/AboutFDA/WhatWeDo/History/Origin/default.htm

U.S. Department of Agriculture. (May 15, 2006). *Celebrating 100 years of FMIA*. Retrieved from http://www.fsis.usda.gov/100years

12 Disaster Preparedness and Response

Disasters—natural or man-made—can have devastating consequences for public health. A breakdown in the water supply can lead to epidemics of waterborne illnesses. Close quarters in shelters can encourage the spread of communicable diseases. People who have lost their homes, possessions, and livelihoods face high levels of emotional stress that challenge their ability to cope.

The events of September 11, 2001, brought home the fact that terrorist attacks could occur on U.S. soil, and many preparedness programs were started as a direct result. In 2005, hurricane Katrina showed that there were still tremendous gaps in our nation's ability to respond to a public health disaster. Research and planning to ensure a thorough, rapid response to another such emergency continue to this day.

Today, many public health professionals consider disaster preparedness to be part of their jobs. No matter what their primary responsibilities are, health department employees participate in preparedness trainings and drills. Public health responsibilities after a disaster include ensuring availability of essential health care services, monitoring water and sanitation, controlling disease transmission, addressing injury prevention, alerting the public to health concerns, and seeing that vulnerable populations, such as the elderly and the disabled, receive the services they need. Some experts use their skills to help manage the aftermath of disasters around the world.

There are researchers studying the physical elements of disasters— from disease vectors to the potential for bioterrorism—and the human response. There are experts helping to organize hospitals, EMS systems, and individual doctors' offices, and others who are working on the best ways to handle chemical spills or nuclear radiation. Some experts are involved in planning communication networks and data collection systems to allow rapid assessment of public health needs. There are many opportunities in all areas of public health.

This chapter offers a sampling of the jobs in public health preparedness. Many of the people profiled in other chapters also mentioned disaster planning among their responsibilities. The list of specific jobs that could focus on preparedness is too long to include here—but as you look through this book, think about the needs associated with the subject of each chapter. There are disaster preparedness experts working in all of these fields.

EMERGENCY PREPAREDNESS SPECIALIST

Job Description

An emergency preparedness specialist (or "emergency response" or "emergency management" specialist) identifies potential emergencies, draws up plans for government and health care institutions to respond, and ensures that everyone involved is aware of their role if an emergency should occur. Emergency management specialists working in health departments and in other public health roles settings make sure that needed supplies such as food, water, and medical equipment are in place, or that health, safety, and sanitation service teams are prepared to respond. They write or approve manuals and emergency preparedness plans and make sure that the plans comply with national regulations and take advantage of available assistance. Often, they plan and run practice drills and exercises. They communicate and coordinate with other agencies involved in responding to major emergencies. They may inspect facilities that will be part of disaster response and ensure that communication systems are in place and that workers are properly trained. If an emergency occurs, they alert health care providers, public health professionals, or people involved in other vital services and help coordinate the response.

EDUCATION AND CERTIFICATION

A bachelor's degree is usually the minimum qualification, often with education or experience in public administration, public health, social work, or a related field. Because health-related emergency response requires knowledge of the health care fields and the needs of doctors and patients, an MPH or a background in nursing, medicine, or pharmacy can be helpful.

Core Competencies and Skills

- Excellent organizational and managerial skills
- Ability to remain calm under pressure and to keep others calm
- Ability to make decisions independently
- Good communication and presentation skills
- Awareness of news events and current risks
- Ability to work with people of different educational backgrounds and responsibility levels
- Knowledge of state and federal programs and regulations for emergency response

Compensation

The median wage for an emergency management specialist is about $50,000 per year, with most earning between $28,000 and $85,000. Regional directors and high-level directors of emergency management programs can earn more.

Workplaces

Emergency management specialists work at all levels of the public health system and in all the areas of public health. They are found at local and state health departments, as well as federal government agencies. Some work with consulting firms or nonprofit organizations. Hospitals often have coordinators for emergency management. Some corporations also employ specialists to plan the company's response to emergencies, focusing on keeping employees safe or protecting the community from events like chemical spills or nuclear power plant meltdowns.

Employment Outlook

Opportunities for emergency response specialists are expected to expand over the next several years because of concerns about terrorism and an increasing appreciation for the importance of planning for possible disasters.

For Further Information

- National Emergency Management Association (NEMA) *nemaweb.org*
- International Association of Emergency Managers (IAEM) *www.iaem.com*

PUBLIC HEALTH PROFILE: Emergency Preparedness Specialist
Bindy Crouch, MD, MPH
Primary Care Emergency Preparedness Medical Coordinator
New York City Department of Health and Mental Hygiene,
New York, NY

Describe the sort of work you do.

I coordinate emergency preparedness within the primary care community of New York City. For the most part that means outpatient facilities, including the federally qualified health centers, some hospital-affiliated outpatient centers, and some private networks. We help the facilities do internal preparation and build capacity so that they can withstand a disaster on their own, and also be part of the New York City plan for public health emergencies. The types of emergencies we prepare for include pandemic influenza, outbreaks due to bioterrorism agents, emergencies due to hazardous materials, and even a nuclear bomb blast.

What is a typical day like at your job?

I spend about 60% of my time in the office and maybe 30% to 40% doing fieldwork. On a typical office day, a lot of my work is related

Continued

to managing grants. On nonoffice days, I try to get out into the community. I might go to see how a health center is set up and how they are planning to separate infected and noninfected clients during an infectious disease outbreak.

I do a lot of coordinating with other city agencies. I relay information about what capacity the outpatient sites have, where they are, and what roles they could fulfill during an emergency. And I answer questions from the sites and talk with them about how pieces of the plans will be implemented.

My work also includes planning for antiviral distribution from the strategic national stockpile. With the H1N1 flu, I've been managing the process of getting vaccines to sites. Every other month, I also serve as "doctor of the week." For 1 week, I take calls from medical providers about infectious diseases, answer questions, and provide guidance about infection control and outbreak prevention.

What education or training do you have? Is it typical for your job?

Because this is a senior staff position, you have to be a licensed physician and board certified in at least one specialty. I have a medical degree, and I've completed residency training in family medicine and in preventive medicine, which includes an MPH. You could do some of this work without being a doctor, but you'd probably have a doctor overseeing everything you do.

What path did you take to get to the job you are in today?

I worked part-time as a family physician while I was training in preventive medicine. This was my first job after completing my training. I applied for several different positions through the Department of Health Web site, and I worked with the recruiter at the Department. I kept calling them on a regular basis and saying, "I applied for these positions, have you heard anything?"

Continued

Where might you go from here, if you wanted to advance your career?

I'm pretty happy with my level right now. At a health department, doctors usually come in as senior staff, and there aren't that many gradations after that. The next level would be medical director of our program—but there are just a handful of positions at that level. Another option would be to stay at this level but move to a different subject, a different area of public health.

What is the worst or most challenging part of your job?

There are some aspects of managing grants I don't like, like bugging people to get things in on time. Also, working within a huge bureaucracy, it can be difficult to get simple things done quickly.

What is the best part?

I am in a really good learning environment. In New York City there are so many other physicians and PhDs that even though it's government work, there is an element of academia. There is research going on, there are opportunities to speak at grand rounds, and there are weekly meetings to review cases.

What advice do you have for someone who is interested in your career?

An important decision to make is what role you want to play. Do you want to be managing people and programs? Do you want to be "boots on the ground" and doing the work yourself? I'm in a management job, and that's about the level you come in at here if you're a physician. If you have visions of going out and giving people their TB medications every day, that's most typically not a physician's role. I think that how much you'll enjoy the job has much less to do with what the subject matter is and more to do with what kind of work you want to do.

ENVIRONMENTAL HEALTH EMERGENCY RESPONSE SPECIALIST

Job Description

Some environmental health experts focus on handling environmental emergencies, such as hazardous waste spills, industrial fires, radiological emergencies, or chemical attacks, or on responding to major disruptions in water and sanitation services. Specific jobs vary, as the role for an environmental health expert in emergency preparedness is still an emerging one. In general, these experts identify hazards, assist with plans for hazard control, and determine what type of emergency response would be needed in a given situation. They may map out areas that are particularly vulnerable and pinpoint areas where response capability should be increased. They might be charged with drawing up or contributing to protocols for assessing potentially contaminated air, food, and water, or for the decontamination of people and of the environment. They may help predict the contamination patterns that would occur with certain events and conditions and determine whether contamination levels are likely to pose health concerns. Some are involved in ensuring that government agencies and outside partners comply with regulations related to hazard control and preparedness. When outside companies are tasked with completing certain jobs, they make sure the work is done appropriately and on time. Conducting trainings and presenting information to staff members are also typical responsibilities.

Environmental preparedness experts work primarily during regular business hours—but when an emergency does happen, these experts may be called upon to respond.

Education and Certification

Educational requirements vary. There are jobs for registered sanitarians, for those with bachelor's or master's degrees in environmental health or in chemistry, biology, or physics, and even for doctoral-level scientists. Entry-level opportunities may require basic technical knowledge and the ability to complete straightforward assessments; more complex jobs require more extensive knowledge and often management or research experience.

Core Competencies and Skills

- Ability to work on a team with other public health professionals
- Knowledge of environmental risks to health and how to control or mitigate them
- Understanding of local and national preparedness efforts
- Understanding of epidemiology
- Knowledge of how to assess environmental contamination and related health risks
- Awareness of laws and regulations pertaining to preparedness and response

Compensation

There is a wide range of salaries, depending on the specifications of the job and the training and experience required. One environmental protection assistant job with the federal government has a salary range of $37,000 to $53,000. A job for an environmental scientist who forecasts the effects of disasters involving the water supply pays $51,000 to $81,000. An environmental scientist doing preparedness work with a major city's health department can earn nearly $100,000 per year.

Workplaces

There are environmental health experts working on emergency preparedness at local and state health departments, at state environmental agencies, and at other departments concerned with preparedness and health. At the federal level, there are opportunities at the EPA, the CDC, the Department of the Interior, and other agencies. There are also opportunities in industry to contribute to environmental preparedness; for example, an industrial hygienist's job may include preparing for chemical fires, spills, or other emergencies.

Employment Outlook

Environmental emergencies may be grouped with other potential public health emergencies or with general safety concerning toxic substances used in industry, which means that it may be challenging to find job listings specifically for environmental preparedness. In general, however, there is a demand for people who are knowledgeable about a wide range of issues in emergency management, including environmental concerns.

For Further Information

- National Environmental Health Association—Terrorism and All-Hazards Preparedness Program
  www.neha.org/preparedness
- American Industrial Hygiene Association—Incident Preparedness and Response Working Group
  www.aiha.org/insideaiha/volunteergroups/Pages/IncidentPreparedness.aspx

DISASTER PREPAREDNESS RESEARCHER

Job Description

Public health planning for an emergency or disaster requires an understanding of how people are likely to behave and what they will need on both the physical and psychological levels. Providing such knowledge is the job of researchers who focus on disaster preparedness. These scientists study issues such as psychological responses to disasters, ways to help people remain calm, and procedures and programs that are most likely to gain the public's cooperation and prevent chaos. For example, if you recommend that people "shelter in place" (staying home rather than going to a central location), will they listen? Will doctors, firefighters, and ambulance personnel report to work, or will they stay home to try to protect their families? How can technology help keep people informed during a disaster?

Disaster preparedness researchers also share what they have learned with legislators and government officials, and they work to ensure that the knowledge they gather is actually used. The job usually combines deskwork with some degree of fieldwork or clinical research, which can include community visits and even international travel.

Education and Certification

Being in charge of this type of research generally requires a PhD or other doctoral-level degree in a medical, social science, or public health field. A master's degree, such as an MPH, or bachelor's degree will suffice for those who want to assist with the research. In some cases, people with master's degrees can also find work designing and carrying out their own studies.

Core Competencies and Skills

- Interest in problem solving and detective work
- Initiative and ability to see projects through to the end
- Good leadership skills
- Good verbal and written communication skills
- Understanding of human psychology and an appreciation for cultural differences
- Understanding of epidemiology and statistics, and the principles of designing and conducting research studies
- Awareness of current knowledge in emergency planning and the public's reactions

Compensation

Many people who do disaster preparedness research are university faculty. According to the 2008 to 2009 salary survey by the American Association of University Professors, the average salary for professors of any rank at institutions granting a significant number of doctoral degrees was $90,055; full professors earned an average of $123,785. Salaries were lower at schools focusing on master's or baccalaureate degrees. Faculty at private universities tend to earn more than those at public ones, and salaries are often higher in urban areas.

Workplaces

Researchers in the public health aspect of emergency preparedness are often based at universities, including schools of public health.

Employment Outlook

This is a specialized field, and there is a limited number of job openings. At the same time, however, there are a limited number of people who are interested in or qualified to do this type of work. Competition for jobs will depend on trends in government funding and in the decisions that today's degree candidates make about the direction of their work. Also, many current job openings are for accomplished scientists; a new graduate who does not find an immediate opening may be able to begin with a job in a related field, then look for appropriate grants and work toward making this a focus of his or her studies.

For Further Information

There is no single association for disaster preparedness researchers. However, these may be helpful:

- Columbia University's National Center for Disaster Preparedness (NCDP) *www.ncdp.mailman.columbia.edu*
- Natural Hazards Center at the University of Colorado, Boulder *www.colorado.edu/hazard*
- Disaster Research Center (DRC), University of Delaware *www.udel.edu/DRC*

PUBLIC HEALTH PROFILE: Disaster Preparedness Researcher
David Abramson, PhD
Director of Research
National Center for Disaster Preparedness
Columbia University Mailman School of Public Health, New York, NY

Describe the sort of work you do.

The National Center for Disaster Preparedness (NCDP) is a multidisciplinary academic center within the Mailman School of Public Health. We do public health research related to disaster preparedness, response, and recovery. We look at the health consequences of an event and ask, "What are the problems that can occur? How can they be prevented?" We think about the effects of policy, system readiness and interorganizational relationships, and the impact of disasters on vulnerable populations. We consider solutions that can occur at the individual, community, or organizational level, all the way up to federal policy.

What is a typical day like at your job?

On any given day, I spend at least some of my time managing my research projects. That could mean running focus groups, speaking with assistants who are out in the field collecting data, or looking at the best way to make a research operation run. If I want to send 20 people to the Gulf Coast, I have to plan how to do that.

Continued

My days also include thinking about research questions and designing studies to answer those questions. For example, we know that people are generally not physically or emotionally prepared for disasters. My team and I have a hypothesis that people who have taken cardiopulmonary resuscitation (CPR) classes are more likely to be prepared—not just to do CPR, but to evaluate their environment, to make good decisions, and to help others in an emergency. If that's the case, it could be because the types of people who take a CPR class are themselves more likely to be prepared or because the class itself has had some effect. We need to figure out how to design a study to explore this.

Often, I spend part of the day writing up study results or writing grant applications. And part of the day is administrative. There are about 15 people working here, and many report to me. There are a lot of meetings, too—with staff here and with external parties such as government officials, funders, and subject matter experts.

What education or training do you have? Is it typical for your job?

I have a PhD and an MPH. The PhD is in sociomedical sciences, which in my case involved doctoral work in both public health and political science. I also have a BA in English, and I'm a former paramedic. To serve as primary investigator on the types of studies we do at NCDP, you generally need a doctoral-level degree.

What path did you take to get to the job you are in today?

When I was in my 20s, I was a journalist writing for national magazines, including *Rolling Stone* and *Esquire*. I lived in a rural area, and I joined a volunteer ambulance corps just as something to do for the community. To work on the ambulances, I became certified as an emergency medical technician (EMT). Then, I wrote an article on trauma care in the United States, which allowed me to travel around the country and hang out with paramedics. And I thought, this is even better than being an EMT. I trained as a paramedic and thought about going to medical school, but I decided an MPH would be a better fit.

Continued

I wanted to do my own research, and so after the MPH, I started working on my PhD. Shortly after I finished my PhD, I pitched an idea for a disaster-related research project to the director of NCDP. He liked it, and eventually he invited me to join the Center.

Where might you go from here, if you wanted to advance your career?

As faculty, I could work toward becoming a full professor and eventually a center director. Personally, I think my career may loop back to writing. I see the progression being toward writing books, a blend of popular and scientific writing. I could see doing a half writing and half research and teaching role.

What is the worst or most challenging part of your job?

I'm not fond of administrative minutiae and bureaucracy. Often, guidelines for submitting a grant proposal to the NIH or the CDC are filled with what seem like silly, stupid, or arcane rules. More often than not, it seems like a barrier to the work you want to do.

What is the best part?

My favorite part is thinking about a question and coming up with a study design to answer it. It's that whole formative process of getting the thoughts together, getting the people together, and building the teams. There are a million things to think about and it's very intellectually stimulating. The teamwork aspect is fun too. After years of being a solitary writer, going for days without talking to anyone—the camaraderie is terrific.

What advice do you have for someone who is interested in your career?

If you are not a very curious person, this is not the career for you. If you're never satisfied with what you read as being "the answer," then it's a career to consider. You also have to feel there is something fundamentally important about research. You have to be committed to the concept that research is a reasonable and laudable thing to be doing, and that it adds to the good of society.

BIOTERRORISM RESEARCHER

Job Description

Bioterrorism researchers are involved in preparing for the possibility—hopefully remote, but still very real—of a bioterrorism attack. This type of preparedness requires understanding what pathogens or toxins could be used against a population, how tools to diagnose a new disease can be developed *fast*, whether vaccines can be developed, what can be done to ward off biologically based toxins or minimize their effects, and so on. Some of the research is highly practical, whereas some is designed to improve the base of knowledge for future work. Much of this research involves cellular- or molecular-level work using sophisticated equipment. Some researchers do animal studies. As researchers advance through their careers, they may move from doing hands-on work to leading laboratory teams. In most cases, applying for funding to support the research is also part of the job.

Education and Certification

This type of research almost always requires a PhD. Typical areas of expertise include microbiology, virology, bacteriology, immunology, biochemistry, and molecular genetics. Some researchers also have MDs, DVMs, or other clinical degrees. Some have pursued public health training, such as an MPH, in addition to the doctoral degree.

Core Competencies and Skills

- Interest in "hard science" and laboratory research
- Willingness to work nontraditional hours if the research requires
- Ability to think creatively and devise innovative solutions to problems
- Interest in collaborating with other experts to share knowledge and ideas
- Experience with designing studies, carrying them out, and interpreting the results
- Knowledge of cellular and molecular mechanisms of infectious diseases and biologic toxins, as well as their effects on the body as a whole

Compensation

Salaries for researchers focusing on biodefense depend upon experience, location, and specialty. A typical range for faculty in the biological sciences, according to the Bureau of Labor Statistics, is $38,000 to $148,000, with about 10% earning less and 10% earning more. As with other types of laboratory research, new PhDs doing postdoctoral work start at lower salaries, whereas directors of research centers are at the top of the scale.

Workplaces

The NIH supports several regional Centers of Excellence for Biodefense and Emerging Infectious Diseases Research, which bring together researchers from universities and research centers around the region. Scientists who do this type of research are often employed at universities but can also be found at medical centers, nonprofit research institutes, government-run laboratories, and other places where basic research is carried out. There are also opportunities in the federal government, including the military.

Employment Outlook

There has been a recent influx of funding for biodefense research, and interest in the many aspects of preparedness has been strong. Future opportunities will depend largely on the availability of government funding, as well as on the number of new PhDs interested in this type of work.

For Further Information

An Internet search for Centers of Excellence for Biodefense and Emerging Infectious Diseases Research will yield links to the many university departments where this type of work is carried out. See also:

- National Institute of Allergy and Infectious Diseases (NIAID)—Biodefense
  www3.niaid.nih.gov/topics/BiodefenseRelated/Biodefense/default.htm
- Centers for Disease Control and Prevention—Emergency Preparedness and Response/Bioterrorism
  www.bt.cdc.gov/bioterrorism

REFERENCE

Landesman, L. Y. (2006). *Public health management of disasters: The pocket guide.* Washington, DC: American Public Health Association.

13   Health Communication

Communication is an essential part of public health work. Health departments and government agencies need to be able to share information with the public and with doctors and other clinicians. Within the public health system, different offices and agencies need to be aware of changes in regulations and policies. Research findings must be disseminated to have an impact.

Sometimes, public health communication is urgent. Citizens need to know when a water purification plant has problems and if they must boil water before drinking it. Doctors need to know if a batch of vaccines is contaminated. And when there are public health scares—a rumor about a contagious disease, for example—people need to know the facts before fears get out of hand.

Other types of communication are planned in advance to address public health issues. There are public campaigns to promote exercise, healthful eating, condom use, HIV testing, and other choices that prevent disease and promote good health. And there are day-to-day outreach efforts to keep important issues in the public's consciousness or remind them of an organization's role. These campaigns may be carried out by local or federal agencies, or by outside organizations concerned with the public's health.

Then there are the research reports, policy papers, regulations, and myriad other documents that circulate among public health professionals, the people who collaborate with them, and the legislators and other stakeholders whose cooperation is essential. Many of these documents are written by researchers or policymakers, but others are created by experts in public health communication. They gather the information and present it in a format and style that match the intended audience.

This chapter has some typical jobs in public health communication. Several other careers in this book may include heavy communications responsibilities; these include medical officer, veterinarian, health promotion coordinator, medical epidemiologist, injury prevention specialist, community activist, nutrition consultant, consumer safety officer, emergency preparedness specialist, advocacy director, policy analyst, grant writer, and the several different researchers.

JOURNALIST

Job Description

Is journalism really a part of public health? It can be. The media is a major source of health information. Newspapers and magazines run regular stories about health issues, and television news often includes a daily health segment. Health journalists are specifically trained to report on these kinds of stories. They give people information that they need to stay healthy. A health journalist with an interest in promoting public health can seek out opportunities to investigate food contamination hazards, expose dangerous practices at a factory, explain how to avoid infectious or chronic diseases, and correct myths and misunderstandings. He can also focus on policy, such as helping the public to understand discussions of health system reform.

Journalists divide their time among gathering information by phone and online, conducting telephone interviews with experts, participating in press briefings, attending hearings and events, and writing their articles or reports. Television reporters may do on-site reporting at medical centers and laboratories. Investigations may take reporters all over the country or even the world, and health reporters are often called to the scene after hurricanes, earthquakes, and other disasters that require a public health response. In today's media world, reporters may also need to be able to write stories geared toward the Internet, take their own photos, and even shoot and edit video.

Education and Certification

A bachelor's degree in journalism or mass communications, with classes in science or health reporting, is the most straightforward path to a medical journalism career. A degree in another subject can also be acceptable, if it is combined with experience such as writing for a high-quality college newspaper or interning at a newspaper or television news program. A master's degree provides additional training, makes a candidate more appealing to employers, and can offer entree into the field for those who have an undergraduate degree in a different subject. Any journalist can find himself writing health-related stories, but some master's degree programs allow a focus on health reporting. Some schools offer a master's degree specifically in health journalism. Multimedia skills can also be useful.

Core Competencies and Skills

- Superb written and spoken communication skills
- Basic understanding of biology, medicine, and public health issues
- High level of comfort with "cold-calling" experts, patients, company executives, and other people who are strangers to you
- Good interpersonal skills
- High level of integrity
- Ability to work under pressure and to meet tight deadlines
- Ability to tell a story in different ways for different audiences
- Understanding of what facts are important and of what will be interesting to readers

Compensation

It is difficult to find salary information specifically for health journalists, but in 2008 the median salary for reporters in general was $34,000 per year. Most earned between $20,000 and $77,000. Top journalists can earn $100,000 and more.

Workplaces

Journalists work for newspapers, television stations and networks, Web sites, and other media outlets. Typically, staff reporters cover multiple beats, not just medicine and public health. There are also many freelancers who come up with story ideas, pitch them to editors, complete the assignments they receive, and send out their own invoices for payment.

Employment Outlook

Journalism jobs are constantly in demand, because people tend to think of them as glamorous and exciting. A combination of training, talent, persistence, and patience is the best route to landing a health journalism job. Agreeing to intern at a newspaper or television station is often a good way "in." In recent years, the Internet has radically changed the way people use media, and job prospects for journalists have been on the decline. However, there are still a limited number of people with strong skills in health and science reporting, so opportunities are better in those areas. Today's journalists often cobble together multiple types of work—from news reporting to writing for foundations or niche publications—to create a career.

For Further Information

- Association of Health Care Journalists (AHCJ)
  www.healthjournalism.org
- National Association of Medical Communicators (NAMC)
  www.namc.info

COMMUNICATIONS DIRECTOR

Job Description

A communications director (also sometimes called a public relations director or director of public affairs) manages the interface between a corporation, government agency, or nonprofit organization and the outside world. It is this person's job to ensure that communication with the public or news media is accurate, timely, and clear. Communications directors also aim to put the organization in the best possible light and to further its goals. There are many opportunities for communications professionals in public health. Government agencies and nonprofit organizations have communications teams to field questions from reporters, connect journalists to the most appropriate experts, and prepare fact sheets, press releases, and information updates that reporters can use. In small organizations, the director may also carry out most of the work; in large ones, he or she oversees a staff. At a health department, the communications director helps control what information is released in case of an outbreak or epidemic. He or she is also in charge of managing any public concerns or criticisms about the organization and its work.

This is generally an office job with standard hours, but when events are scheduled, emergencies happen, or important campaigns are launched, weekend work and late evenings can become the norm. Outside meetings and travel may also be important elements of the job.

Education and Certification

A communications director needs at least a bachelor's degree, and a master's degree may be preferred. Typical subjects are communications, journalism, public relations, and marketing. Often, a degree in a field that matches the agency's or organization's interests is also acceptable. Communications professionals generally start in lower-level jobs and work their way up to higher-level positions; a communications director usually needs at least several years of experience. No special certifications are required, but voluntary certifications are available, such as the Accredited in Public Relations designation through the Public Relations Society of America.

Core Competencies and Skills

- Excellent written and spoken communication skills
- Good time management and organizational skills, to help reporters meet deadlines
- Knowledge of public health issues important to the agency or organization
- Understanding of the needs of reporters, bloggers, and others who share information with the public
- Understanding of marketing principles, including how to plan a campaign and evaluate its success
- Ability to write a press release and prepare other materials for reporters to use
- Good sense for business strategy and for planning toward long-

range goals
- Good interpersonal skills and initiative to develop connections with reporters, other media professionals, and experts

Compensation

For public relations specialists in general, the median salary in 2008 was $51,000, with most earning between $30,000 and $98,000. The median salary for a public relations manager was about $89,000, with the top 25% earning $126,000 or more. Salaries at nonprofits are often lower than in industry, and some communications directors choose to accept these smaller salaries to work for causes and organizations they believe in.

Workplaces

Just about every large company, nonprofit, and government agency has a communications director. Communications specialists who are interested in public health can be found at local and state health departments, federal agencies involved in health or safety, and nonprofits devoted to specific health issues or focusing on the quality and availability of health care.

Employment Outlook

There is likely to be growth in the public relations job market. However, like jobs in journalism and advertising, these tend to be competitive positions because people think of them as exciting, creative, and even fun. It can be hard to find a job in a specific agency or subject area, so it is often a good idea to accept a job in a related area, get some experience, and then watch for other openings. Starting with an unpaid internship can be a good way to get experience and make connections, too.

For Further Information

- Public Relations Society of America (PRSA)
  www.prsa.org
- The Association for Women in Communications (AWC)
  www.womcom.org

PUBLIC HEALTH PROFILE: Communications Director Katherine Hull

Vice President of Communications

Rape, Abuse and Incest National Network, Washington, DC

Describe the sort of work you do.

I handle communications for the Rape, Abuse and Incest National Network (RAINN), a national nonprofit dedicated to preventing sexual violence and helping victims of rape and abuse. This is an enormously important issue: 1 in 6 women and 1 in 33 men in the United States will be sexually assaulted in their lifetimes, and victims are at increased risk of depression, substance abuse, and even suicide. RAINN addresses these issues on a population level by operating a national telephone and online hotline, educating the public, and working toward improving policy. At the communications department, we promote the work of RAINN to the public through a variety of different means. That includes public relations, marketing, social networking, and even working with members of the entertainment industry.

What is a typical day like at your job?

A main aspect of my job is working with the media, which is a balance between proactive and reactive interactions. Proactively, I'll contact specific reporters when we have a story that I think they will be interested in—and reactively, I'll help reporters who call for information on stories they are working on. I also look for ways that RAINN can contribute to a breaking story. For instance, when a celebrity recently disclosed her experience with being sexually absued as a child, we were able to work with key reporters to talk about the impact on Americans, as demonstrated by the large number of calls to our hotlines. We transformed the media coverage from a story about just one celebrity to a story about how a celebrity inspired thousands of people to reach out for help.

As the organization's spokesperson, I sometimes participate in radio or television talk shows. We also work with the entertainment industry on their depictions of sexual violence. In one of my favorite experiences, I helped the writers of a soap opera craft a scene accurately depicting the aftermath of a sexual assault, to teach viewers how to preserve forensic evidence and report to police. Another aspect

Continued

of my job is working with our celebrity supporters. I'll coordinate with publicists and brief celebrities before events or media interviews.

Some of my other responsibilities are managing the organization's website and social networking presence, overseeing our newsletter, and writing press releases.

What education or training do you have? Is it typical for your job?

You don't necessarily need a degree in communications to do this type of work. My bachelor's degree is in political science and history. Many people at my level have a bachelor's or a master's degree.

What path did you take to get to the job you are in today?

I moved to Washington, DC, because I wanted to get involved in politics. My first position was an internship on Capitol Hill for a senator. It was a fabulous experience, but it left me with a desire to explore other areas of work. I took a job with a public affairs firm where I gained experience in crisis management while working for the firm's client base of large for-profit companies. I learned more about communications and the media, and the importance not just of doing good work, but of telling people about it. I realized that I wanted to help a good nonprofit organization tell its story. A friend sent me the job posting from RAINN.

Where might you go from here, if you wanted to advance your career?

I'm constantly setting new goals, finding new partnerships and new ways to reach out to our target audience, so every day is different and exciting. In my current position, I head up the department, so I suppose if I wanted to make a change, the next step would be working for a larger organization. Knowing how to tell the story behind an organization or company is a valuable skill set that could translate to any issue.

What is the worst or most challenging part of your job?

It's frustrating when a reporter omits information I've pushed for in a piece. For example, there have been times when I've invested a lot of time with a reporter on a specific story, only to find that a mention of

Continued

our organization didn't make the final cut. Sometimes it is not even the reporter's fault—the editor makes the cut. At the end of the day, you can't let it bother you too much. It is just part of the job.

What is the best part?

I really enjoy working with the entertainment industry and working with TV show writers on plot lines related to our issues. I also love having the flexibility to pursue goals that further the organization's mission and on a personal level, feel challenged on a daily basis. It can be difficult to hear stories of people who have suffered, but what gets me through the day is knowing that the work we are doing is helping people turn their lives around.

What advice do you have for someone who is interested in your career?

Determine what you're passionate about. When you read the news and look at advertisements, notice what topics you're drawn to, and from there look for jobs in a related field. For nonprofit positions, look for job postings in places where companies can place ads for free, because a lot of nonprofits don't have the resources to pay for ads. As you're applying for jobs, remember that details matter! Spell-check your resume, don't leave in the track-changes notes, and ensure that the cover letter is geared toward the organization you are applying to.

SOCIAL MARKETER

Job Description

Social marketing is a relatively new concept in the United States, although social marketing practices have been used by international health organizations for many years. Social marketing firms and departments use the same techniques and concepts that advertisers use to sell televisions, fast food, and new cars—but they use them to sell healthy behaviors, instead. A social marketing team usually begins with an established need, such as convincing young adult men to be tested for HIV. They do marketing research to figure out what appeals to the population in question. Do these men watch television? Are they likely to pay attention to cell phone text messages? Next, the team comes up with slogans, scripts or ad copy, sample text messages, and so on. They test them with members of the population; then they create final versions and launch the campaign. Afterward, they track the response through surveys, data on web page views, and other measurement techniques. Often, a social marketing expert must figure out how to help an organization accomplish a big goal on a very modest budget. (Make sure not to confuse social marketing with social media marketing, which uses online communities, blogs, and social networks like Twitter to sell products.)

Social marketing agencies work for many different clients and on many different topics. Some organizations have in-house social marketing departments focusing just on their own causes. The job itself is largely office-based but can include conducting focus groups, collaborating with community organizations, attending video shoots, and other outside meetings and events. There may also be travel to meet with clients.

Education and Certification

Because social marketing is an emerging field, there is no single set of qualifications. An MPH, a degree in communications, marketing, or journalism, a background in psychology or another social science, or a background in advertising can all be appropriate. Training or experience in marketing and advertising is helpful. A few schools do now offer graduate-level training in public health marketing, such as an MPH with a social marketing focus or a certificate in public health communication and marketing.

Core Competencies and Skills

- Excellent written and spoken communication skills
- Creativity
- Awareness of current social trends and fads, or the ability to find out
- Appreciation of diversity, including the fact that different community groups have different priorities
- Strong understanding of marketing and media, including how to place ads, gain reporters' attention, and appeal to the general public
- Ability to meet deadlines
- Understanding of how to present information for people with low health literacy
- Knowledge of survey and evaluation techniques

Compensation

Salaries for people involved in social marketing will vary depending on the type of organization, the amount of funding available, and the scope of the work. A starting salary in the $40,000 to $50,000 range would not be unusual, with higher salaries for people with more experience and responsibility.

Workplaces

Many people involved in social marketing work for independent firms that offer their services to health-oriented nonprofits and government agencies. Some of these are respected advertising or consulting agencies, while others are small start-ups with just a few clients. Other people involved in this field work directly for government agencies or for nonprofit organizations that focus on specific health issues.

Employment Outlook

Awareness of social marketing seems to be increasing, but many people in American public health are still either unaware of this discipline or uncertain about what the term means. On the other hand, this means that a creative, ambitious person has the opportunity to blaze new trails, such as helping to start a company or create a new department. Overall, opportunities will depend on interest from government and nonprofits and on the funding available. One way to get a toehold in this field is to begin with an internship at a social marketing firm; another is to begin with a job in communications or community outreach that incorporates some social marketing efforts.

For Further Information

- You can learn about social marketing campaigns by visiting companies' Web sites and looking at their work.
- American Marketing Association (AMA)
  www.marketingpower.com
- CDC's National Center for Health Marketing
  www.cdc.gov/healthmarketing
- The Ad Council
  www.adcouncil.org

PUBLIC HEALTH PROFILE: Social Marketer
Les Pappas
President and Creative Director
Better World Advertising, San Francisco, CA/New York, NY

Describe the sort of work you do.

I own an agency that does social marketing with a focus on health and social issues. We work closely with clients to make the most effective use of their resources. We do needs assessments, help clients understand how to get a message out, develop campaigns and interventions, and evaluate the effects of our campaigns. We work in all communication vehicles, including television, radio, print, and billboards, and we're doing more and more on the Internet. We do most of the creative work in-house and also hire photographers and illustrators and other help as needed.

We've done campaigns on many topics, and each one requires its own approach. Doing suicide prevention with teens is very different than trying to get adults to stop smoking. Right now I'm doing an AIDS prevention project in Indonesia. The setting, culture, values—everything has to be taken into account.

What is a typical day like at your job?

As the president and creative director, I have a hand in just about everything. A typical day could involve working with our designers on developing concepts for ads, writing copy for brochures, facilitating focus groups, and doing media buys and strategies. Yesterday, I was talking to a cable company about adjusting the time slots for some commercials, and then I was writing proposals to potential clients for some web and brochure work. I write and edit reports on focus groups, I write recommendations for clients on what we advise for campaigns, and I create annual reports for clients—lots of writing, editing, and reviewing documents.

I also have a lot of meetings with clients, other stakeholders, and advisors. We have lots of brainstorming sessions, too. The heart and soul of what we do is coming up with ideas and developing concepts for campaigns. And then of course we find the best ways to carry them out.

Continued

What education or training do you have? Is it typical for your job?

I have a bachelor's degree in government and history and an MPA degree. We have people on our staff who have MPHs, people who have experience in advertising, people who have degrees in communications, graphic designers, and artists. This kind of work is generally very collaborative, so it is nice to have people with different backgrounds and different experience.

What path did you take to get to the job you are in today?

I started out working on political campaigns. I worked for Ted Kennedy and for Paul Tsongas in Massachusetts. Then I moved to San Francisco in the early 1980s, at the same time that HIV/AIDS was coming onto the scene. As a gay man, I was very drawn to that issue, and I started working for the San Francisco AIDS Foundation. That's how I got into public health and social marketing. I learned about market research, focus groups, all that sort of thing, in order to do the work we needed to do. Eventually I decided I wanted to expand to other issues, and I wanted to share what I had learned. I started Better World Advertising in 1996.

Where might you go from here, if you wanted to advance your career?

I own the company, so for me the "next step" would have to be pretty impressive. The independence would be very hard to give up. For the people working within the company, there are lots of different career avenues. There are many issue-oriented organizations that have in-house people to work on social marketing, so that would be one option.

What is the worst or most challenging part of your job?

One challenge lies in educating the clients. We're known for creating campaigns that are kind of edgy, that push the envelope. Sometimes

Continued

being controversial or confrontational helps to get people's attention. But clients often work within bureaucratic systems that don't reward taking risks. That means most of the social marketing you see is kind of boring and safe, and we don't do that. We have to educate our clients about the fact that they have to take some risks to get results.

What is the best part?

Before I started doing social marketing, I didn't even know I was a creative person. But I found that I am. It is in the ability to communicate, to come up with ideas, to write copy. I also enjoy having the opportunity to put my ideas out there—that I can be walking down the street and see a bus go by, and my company's ad is on that bus.

What advice do you have for someone who is interested in your career?

You need to be passionate about the issue you are working on, but you also need to have some objectivity and distance to create a good social marketing campaign. The people who do suicide prevention or adoption work or HIV vaccine research are completely immersed in that issue all day every day. I do that for part of my day. You have to have a balance between passion and objectivity.

MEDICAL WRITER

Job Description

Medical writers create informational articles, reports, and educational materials for consumers, health professionals, and public health experts. Their work may appear in magazines, on Web sites, on television and in other media outlets. Or, they may write documents, newsletters, and articles targeted to very specific audiences. Unlike journalists, medical writers generally do not seek out news stories or investigate health claims or questionable practices. Instead, they organize and summarize health information. For example, a medical writer might be behind a series of Web site articles, sponsored by a government agency, offering information for parents about children's health problems. There are medical writers who compose educational materials to keep health professionals up to date about new developments in patient care and public health. Medical writers are also involved in helping researchers craft grant proposals, and some write regulatory documents for government agencies. Medical writers must be able to understand complicated research studies, textbooks, and experts' opinions and present the information in a readable, straightforward, and useful way.

Education and Certification

Some medical writers come from journalism backgrounds. Others have bachelor's or higher degrees in biology, chemistry, or physics. Some are trained as doctors or nurses. People with advanced degrees are common in medical writing—a survey by the American Medical Writers Association (AMWA) found that 43% of people with entry-level jobs had doctoral degrees. Although there is no specific educational pathway to this job, a medical writer must have the knowledge to interpret health information accurately.

Core Competencies and Skills

- Excellent writing skills
- Curiosity about medical and public health issues
- Knack for "translating" information from medical research and complex reports into less difficult language, and for matching the reading level to the audience
- Ability to write in multiple styles
- Understanding of what sort of information doctors, nurses, other professionals, and the general public need to know
- Ability to meet deadlines, which can sometimes be tight

Compensation

According to a 2007 survey of members of AMWA, entry-level salaries for writers with at least a master's degree averaged about $60,000. Salaries for people with strong skills and experience or advanced degrees can range to $100,000 or higher. Writers for government agencies do tend to be at the lower end of the pay scale, compared to those in for-profit industries. Freelancers often earn over $100,000 per year in gross income, although they don't receive employee perks such as paid vacation or health insurance.

Workplaces

In public health, medical writers work for government agencies like the CDC or the USDA, state and local health departments, research organizations, consulting firms, and nonprofits. There are also jobs at Web sites focusing on medical information for the public. Many medical writers are freelancers, taking on specific assignments for various clients. Medical writers can also find work with pharmaceutical companies and other for-profit industries, but these jobs are usually related more to selling products than to directly promoting health.

Employment Outlook

Medical writers are consistently in demand, and in fact the field has expanded greatly in recent years. Breaking into the field can be challenging, however. Writing for smaller organizations and publications, even for free, can be a way to collect some "clips" (sample articles) to show potential employers.

For Further Information

■ American Medical Writers Association (AMWA)
www.amwa.org
■ National Association of Science Writers (NASW)
www.nasw.org

14 Education

This chapter is about the people who ensure that our children learn basic information about health, our public health professionals are prepared for practice, and our doctors, nurses, and dentists are up-to-date. All of these types of education contribute to our nation's capacity for health and safety.

For the general public, lack of basic health knowledge can have serious consequences. Misunderstandings about disease transmission can lead to personal illness—or a citywide epidemic. Myths about sex can lead to HIV infection and other serious infections, as well as unintended pregnancies.

There are educational needs for health professionals, too. The training that they receive when they earn their degrees is just the beginning. Health information can change *fast*, thanks to new discoveries—and if our providers' knowledge is out of date, it becomes a problem for everyone. "Continuing education" classes and activities help health professionals keep their knowledge sharp.

Training for public health professionals is vital, as well. Schools of public health help ensure that the public health professionals are equipped to meet local, national, and global needs. Then also support the research that leads to new innovations.

HEALTH TEACHER

Job Description

Health teachers educate children and teens about their bodies and about healthy choices in areas such as nutrition, personal hygiene, disease prevention, and safe sex. In public schools, they are generally required to follow a set curriculum; some private schools allow teachers to design their own courses. Health teachers sometimes have to avoid certain topics, too—for example, some school districts forbid teaching about contraception. Most schools offer at least some health education and, as of 2006, 75% of states required districts or schools to follow national or state standards.

Health teachers usually teach several classes per day. Depending on the school, they may teach just one age group, or multiple levels. They adapt their lessons to meet the needs of each group of students. In some settings, health teachers work with other teachers in the school to dovetail lessons or to promote school wide health campaigns. Many health teachers serve as physical education (PE) teachers, as well. In addition to classroom time, health teachers spend time preparing their lessons, decorating their classrooms, and grading assignments. They enjoy summers off, although many use that time to earn extra money or take classes to further their own education.

Education and Certification

Public school teachers must be licensed, which requires completing a teacher training program and usually an exam, plus taking continuing education classes to maintain the license. The most straightforward path to becoming a health teacher is to earn a bachelor's or master's degree in health education, in a program specifically designed to lead to teacher certification. For people who are already certified, each state has its own requirements regarding additional training for health teachers. There are alternative paths to licensure to fill certain teacher shortages; these also vary by state and subject. Private schools can generally hire teachers who are not licensed, although they may choose to make it a requirement.

Core Competencies and Skills

- Adaptability
- Good organizational skills

- Good time management skills
- Sense of humor
- Ability to keep kids focused and well-behaved
- Ability to explain complicated information in a way kids can understand
- Knowledge of how to find reliable information in the library and on the Internet

Compensation

The median salary for a teacher in 2008 was about $49,000 per year at the elementary school level, $50,000 at the middle school level, and $51,000 at high schools. Most teachers at elementary through high schools earned between $33,000 and $81,000.

Workplaces

Health teachers work at public and private schools. Middle and elementary schools are most likely to require health education. High schools are most likely to have health education teachers handling required health classes, followed by middle schools.

Employment Outlook

The need for health teachers will vary by location, because it depends on student enrollment and local requirements. Enrollments are expected to increase in the South and West over the next several years, decline in the Northeast, and remain steady in the Midwest. Job prospects for teachers will likely be better in urban and rural areas, compared to suburban districts. Health teachers will find the best prospects in areas with high enrollment and in districts that require health education to be delivered by certified health teachers.

For Further Information

- American Association for Health Education
  www.aahperd.org/AAHE
- American Public Health Association—School Health Education and Services Section
  www.apha.org/membergroups/sections/aphasections/schoolhealth
- American School Health Association (ASHA)
  www.ashaweb.org

PUBLIC HEALTH PROFILE: Health Teacher
Steve Haines, MA
Health and PE Teacher
Newtown Friends School, Newtown, PA

Describe the sort of work you do.

I teach at a private school for children in pre-kindergarten through eighth grade. I cover sixth to eighth grade PE and health, I'm the athletic director, and I coach three sports teams. I also teach a section of eighth grade history. There was no PE or health curriculum when I started here, so I created it, and I add to it constantly. Sixth grade health class covers human development, including puberty, male and female anatomy, pregnancy, and some sex education. In seventh grade, the focus is on nutrition. Eighth grade involves independent student or group research and a lot of class debate. We investigate difficult issues such as abortion, right to die, capital punishment, alcohol and drugs, and even intimate partner violence.

What is a typical day like at your job?

My day starts with homeroom. Then some days I teach two classes, and some days I teach four out of the six periods. I supervise students during lunch, recess, and study hall. I coach after school, too, usually 3 or 4 days a week. I use my free periods to grade tests and papers.

I'm constantly updating my lesson plans with new information and activities. Each health class starts with something to pique my students' interest. I'll look for a short video clip, for example, that pertains to what we'll be learning. And then I give them some information, and then we transition into an activity that they can do. We close with something that provides a practical application, like a change they might consider making in their own lives.

In PE, I try to teach a lot of personal fitness. I'm trying to get the kids to take responsibility for their strength and their core muscle development. When we do team sports, I try to choose ones that kids can do socially, not just at school. I try to set games up so that no

Continued

one's sitting out for very long, and I'm a constant cheerleader for the kids at all levels of fitness.

What education or training do you have? Is it typical for your job?

I attended a private Christian school, and then I went to Philadelphia College of Bible as a double major in bible and PE and health, with a minor in history. My teaching certification is only for private school; if I wanted to teach at a public school, I would need a different certification. I earned a master's degree in history after I started teaching, for my own interest and because I wanted to have options—I couldn't imagine still chasing third graders around at age 50!

What path did you take to get to the job you are in today?

My goal was always to teach PE and health in a private school, and this was my first job after graduating. I had driven by this school for 4 years going to college and never knew what a "Friends School" was. But then when I was looking for a job, I decided to call them. They didn't have anything at the time, but they said to go ahead and send a resume, and I did. And shortly thereafter, a job did open up.

Where might you go from here, if you wanted to advance your career?

A lot of people end up in administration, as division head or as principal. I could see myself doing that, but I don't know that I really want to. Many people find the type of teaching they enjoy and just keep doing that, and that may be what I'll do.

What is the worst or most challenging part of your job?

The kids have all this tech stuff, and educators are thinking that the only way that kids can learn in the 21st century is if we wow them with technology. But I think we're losing content in the process, and I'm disappointed by that. I also think it leads to a failure to hold kids

Continued

accountable. If you forgot your homework, it's going to be online on the class Web site. You're not expected to write it down anymore.

What is the best part?

What I enjoy most about teaching is the relationships I'm able to form with students. I have the opportunity to see these kids grow for 3 years, because I teach them in sixth grade through eighth grade. I see them develop their skills. To me, teaching is about more than the subject itself. I'm helping these kids learn the skills they need to live a successful life.

What advice do you have for someone who is interested in your career?

Decide what age groups you want to work with. If you can, take opportunities during your training to visit schools or classes with age groups you might be interested in. If you think you only want to teach kindergarten through third grade, try to get into that age group when you are student teaching, so you can see for sure if you like it.

CONTINUING EDUCATION COORDINATOR

Job Description

Continuing education is required in many different professions. There are continuing education courses specifically addressing public health topics, such as the H1N1 flu pandemic, guidelines for new vaccines, methods for widespread cancer screening and prevention, and disaster preparedness. Courses providing clinical updates help encourage doctors, nurses, and pharmacists to provide high-quality care. A continuing education coordinator is part of a team that helps get information to the professionals who need it. These organizers take on the day-to-day tasks of connecting with topic experts, working with venues or scheduling space within a medical center, and making sure that online programs are working properly. They keep an eye on deadlines and verify that programs meet national requirements. They handle registration for events, scoring of any tests, and approval of credit for participants. They also help to promote the activities to the appropriate doctors, nurses, or other professionals. Coordinators may be involved in writing grant applications to fund programs, too.

Education and Certification

Some coordinator jobs focus on administrative duties. These generally require a bachelor's degree plus good office skills. Some jobs require a bachelor's or master's degree in a related field, such as public health, nursing, or biomedical sciences.

Core Competencies and Skills

- Ability to multi-task
- Excellent organizational skills and the ability to track elements of a project until it is completed
- Ability to work as a member of a team
- General understanding of educational principles
- Strong sense of ethics, to avoid bias in educational programs
- Knowledge of the requirements for continuing education programs

Compensation

A 2004 to 2005 local survey by the Texas Alliance for Continuing Medical Education found a wide range of salaries for continuing medical education professionals, from under $20,000 to over $70,000. People with the title "coordinator" were likely to earn $40,000 or less, although about 25% earned more. Salaries tended to rise with experience and people with master's degrees were likely to earn more than those with lower-level degrees.

Workplaces

Continuing education coordinators are found at health professions schools and at hospitals and medical centers that provide continuing education programs. There are also many private companies that provide continuing education; these tend to be for-profit companies, and people interested in public health will need to assess the balance of profit versus educational motives.

Employment Outlook

There are no national statistics on job outlook for this particular job title. However, with so many doctors, nurses, and other health professionals needing to meet continuing education requirements, there is an ongoing need for programs.

For Further Information

- Alliance for CME
  www.acme-assn.org
- Society for Academic Continuing Medical Education (SACME)
  www.sacme.org

PROFESSOR, SCHOOL OF PUBLIC HEALTH

Job Description

Schools of public health have professors teaching classes in just about every public health-related topic imaginable. There are courses on health economics, cancer epidemiology, the influence of gender on health, the medical issues that arise in refugee camps, and many other issues. The professors who teach these classes usually have personal experience with the subject matter, either as researchers or through experience in previous careers. They share their expertise with undergraduates, graduate students, or both, depending on the school. They decide what information will be included in a class, assign readings, projects, and papers, and grade their students' work. In large lecture classes they often have help from teaching assistants. Sometimes, professors bring in outside experts to share their experiences, too. Professors often teach two or three classes each semester, with each one taking up a few hours of weekly classroom time plus many more hours in preparation and grading. They may also serve as advisors to individual students working on independent projects. With the rest of their time, they do research, write papers or textbooks, and prepare applications for grants to fund their work. Some offer consulting services to government agencies or businesses, or collaborate with nonprofits and community groups. Professors' research interests may bring them into medical laboratories or clinics, out into the community, and even to exotic locations overseas.

Education and Certification

Becoming a professor at a university usually requires a high-level academic degree, such as a PhD, MD, or DrPH. Some public health professors hold MBAs or JDs. Often, those who were originally trained in a field other than public health have earned MPH degrees, as well.

Core Competencies and Skills

- Patience
- Creativity
- Initiative (to conceive of research projects, find support, and see them through)
- Strong written and spoken communication skills
- Ability to motivate students
- Ability to break information down into manageable segments that people new to a topic can understand
- Deep understanding of one or more aspects of public health, with an interest in learning more

Compensation

Professors usually start at an entry-level job with a title such as "assistant professor." With a strong track record of research and publications, they eventually reach the rank of "full professor." The average salary for faculty of any rank at universities with a significant focus on doctoral-level education was $90,055, based on the 2008 to 2009 salary survey by the American Association of University Professors. Assistant professors earned $70,613 on average and full professors, $123,785.

Workplaces

In addition to schools of public health, professors specializing in public health can be found at medical schools, schools of veterinary medicine, dentistry, and nursing, and university departments focused on related topics such as ecology, sociology, and psychology.

Employment Outlook

Overall, the need for postsecondary teachers—professors and others who teach students who have already completed high school—is expected to expand. At the same time, however, academic jobs, particularly tenure-track jobs, are quite competitive. (Tenure is a designation, based on accomplishment, which guarantees a certain level of job security.) Many colleges and universities have been rethinking how tenure works and are offering fewer-tenure-track positions and more part-time and non-tenure-track positions as a cost-saving measure.

For Further Information

■ Association of Schools of Public Health (ASPH)
www.asph.org

DEAN, SCHOOL OF PUBLIC HEALTH

Job Description

The dean at a school of public health is both an academic and administrative leader. Working with faculty and with other leaders at the university, the dean is instrumental in shaping the school's educational programs, research, and service, and in raising the funds that keep the school running. She also represents the school in the public and professional community. Day-to-day work can include meetings with professors and administrators about educational strategy, discussions about the budget and how the school is funded, conversations with other public health leaders, and events to keep funders aware of the school's plans and accomplishments. The dean provides guidance on what's best for the school and its students, as well as on how the school can maximize its contributions to the science and practice of public health. To do so, she must have extensive knowledge of public health practice and must keep up-to-date on developments in the field. Another important part of the job is knowing how to delegate tasks effectively. A school of public health will generally have assistant or associate deans who oversee specific areas of responsibility, such as financial matters or human resources. This job requires a significant time commitment beyond standard working hours, including evening events and travel to meetings and conferences.

Education and Certification

A dean must be an experienced and accomplished scholar in a public health field. The job requires a terminal academic degree, such as a PhD or DrPH, and significant achievements in research and practice. Institutions look for people who have demonstrated abilities in leadership and strategic planning. The traditional way to become a dean is to begin as a faculty member and rise through the academic ranks. However, people with other types of public health leadership experience can be considered for the job, if they meet the qualifications.

Core Competencies and Skills

- Strong management skills
- Excellent communication skills
- Ability to manage multiple responsibilities and delegate tasks effectively
- Ability not only to get along with diverse faculty members, but to help them get along with each other
- Extensive knowledge of and experience in a public health field
- Understanding of potential funders' interests and of how to connect their interests with those of the school
- Sense of dedication to maintaining high standards, developing effective new programs, and integrating the school with the community and the larger world of public health

Compensation

According to the 2009 to 2010 salary survey by the College and University Professional Association for Human Resources, the median salary for a public health dean was about $272,000. Salaries do vary according to the institution's funding and the individual's qualifications and experience.

Workplaces

This job is found only at universities with schools of public health.

Employment Outlook

The role of dean is open only to particularly accomplished scholars and leaders. There are about 40 to 50 accredited schools of public health in the United States, so the number of openings is extremely limited. Faculty members who are interested in becoming dean of a school of public health should look for opportunities to demonstrate leadership in addition to conducting research, publishing scholarly papers, and maintaining an excellent reputation at the school and in the wider public health world.

For Further Information

■ See the information in the description for professor, school of public health.

PUBLIC HEALTH PROFILE: Dean, School of Public Health
Linda P. Fried, MD, MPH
Dean, Mailman School of Public Health
Columbia University, New York, NY

Describe the sort of work you do.

The Mailman School of Public Health has about 300 full-time faculty and more than 1,000 students. We are dedicated to the development of knowledge that will improve our society, and we have the privilege of creating knowledge that will have an impact not only today but in 20 to 30 years. We translate information and research results into innovative and impactful ways to prevent disability and illness, both for the community and for the use of individual clinicians, and we bring that knowledge to bear in educating future leaders. As dean, my job is to guide the school as we strive to accomplish our mission. It's about finding what will have the most impact and make the most difference.

What is a typical day like at your job?

I come in around 8 or 8:30 a.m., and I'm done in the office around 6:30 or 7 p.m. Then, there is often a meeting in the evening or a dinner with someone to talk about raising funds for the school or other important issues.

There are many things I might do on a typical day. An important part of my day right now is meeting with members of my core team for strategic planning. We've set the goals of the school for the next 5 or 10 years, and we are working hard on implementing a strategy that will allow us to meet those goals. I direct and oversee the shaping this entire effort. I appoint leaders, but I stay engaged and attend the meetings. I'm the guide, the cheerleader, and the coach.

Another big part of my job is finding the resources to accomplish our school's goals. I'm responsible for seeing that the school is in

Continued

good financial shape. I plan the budget, together with the vice dean who is in charge of that. I work with my development office to identify grants we should apply for. I meet with individual philanthropists who might be interested in funding our efforts. I'm also working with an associate dean on improving our research infrastructure, and I'm about to start working with faculty on changes to our curriculum. I serve as the school's representative to the outside world, too, so I talk to reporters, I write articles and op-eds, and I even get involved in public policy. And I meet with students to find out how their educational experiences are going.

What education or training do you have? Is it typical for your job?

I have an MD and an MPH, and I have a great deal of experience in the worlds of public health, geriatrics, science, medicine, and leadership. A dean is usually someone who has had an influential career as a scientist or educator and has already led programs of significance.

What path did you take to get to the job you are in today?

I majored in history and had several jobs before working as a welfare caseworker, which is what sparked my interest in health care. My medical training focused on general internal medicine, geriatrics, and cardiovascular epidemiology. I spent many years as a professor at Johns Hopkins University, where I served as director of multiple research centers and led many studies on aging and health. I'm also a co-founder of Experience Corps, a program that engages older adults to tutor and mentor elementary school students and is also a health promotion program for the older adults. I was elected to the National Institute of Medicine in 2001, and I have participated in many national and international conversations related to issues in gerontology, how we transform well to an aging society, and how to keep all of us healthy. The job of dean is usually offered by invitation, and I was invited to take on the leadership at Mailman.

Continued

Where might you go from here, if you wanted to advance your career?

A dean could go on to be a university president, to lead a foundation, to take a high-level position in a government agency. As for me, I love my job! I could be happy doing this for a long time.

What is the worst or most challenging part of your job?

My workdays can be long, so I would say one of the hardest parts has been learning how to balance a demanding professional life with a fulfilling personal life.

What is the best part?

I care greatly about the issues that I am working on. I also get to be deeply intellectual, and I get to be a scientist at a level that I love. I like thinking about the big picture, how to make a change, and how to lead so that the school achieves the best possible outcomes.

What advice do you have for someone who is interested in your career?

You're smart to think about it, because it's fabulous! I would say to invest in understanding the stages of a career, go in directions that you care about, and try to make a difference. Learn the skills of leadership and management, even if it's not part of your job description. Learn time management, how to handle conflict constructively, and how to set a clear long-term goal. At each stage of your career, look for ways to add to those skills, and think about the next step so you are prepared to move into it.

REFERENCE

Kann, L., Brener N. D., & Wechsler, H. (2007) Overview and summary: School Policies and Programs Study 2006. *Journal of School Health, 77*(8), 385–397.

15

Health Disparities, Vulnerable Groups, and At-Risk Populations

Certain groups are at particularly high risk of health problems compared to the population as a whole. Health disparities between certain ethnic and racial minority groups and White populations are one major concern. There are significant disparities in many types of cancer, diabetes, vaccination rates, infant mortality, and the prevalence and incidence of HIV, for example.

The reasons for many of these disparities aren't completely clear. Causes probably differ from one health problem to another, and from one population to another. Does it have to do with where people live? Their culture or lifestyle? It is an effect of racism? Differences in income or access to care? Public health professionals throughout the country are working to find the answers and to bring our entire population to the same standard of health.

Other types of populations are at elevated risk of certain health problems, too. The elderly, people with physical and/or mental disabilities, people living in poverty, recent immigrants, and refugees are all vulnerable to certain health concerns. Prison inmates are a special population with elevated health risks and a limited ability to control their own care.

In addition to the careers in this chapter, many other public health jobs focus on improving the health of vulnerable groups or incorporate this goal as part of a larger scope of work. They include medical officer, public health nurse, study coordinator, health educator, health promotion coordinator, public health dentist, behavioral scientist, injury prevention specialist, environmental health nurse, community activist, emergency preparedness specialist, social marketer, health teacher, behavioral health program manager, public health social worker, homeless services educator, public health advisor, outcomes researcher, and program officer, as well as several of the jobs in the chapters on health care administration and leadership and maternal and child health.

DIRECTOR, OFFICE OF MINORITY HEALTH

Job Description

Many state health agencies have offices dedicated to alleviating health disparities. The exact names vary, but "Office of Minority Health" is a common variation; other names include "Office of Health Disparities" and "Office of Health Equity." An emerging trend is for city and county health departments to have their own such offices, focusing on local needs. These departments use a combination of activities to accomplish their goals, and they have directors who are closely involved in the day-to-day work. Typically, the work of a county Office of Minority Health will be based on information about the health of different population groups, things like premature births, vaccination coverage, and diabetes prevalence. The director, often working with a small staff, attempts to identify where the disparities are and to begin figuring out why they exist. Then, the office sponsors programs or works with community groups to address the problem. Some of the programs are traditional, but some can be quite creative—like training barbershop staff to talk to their clients about cancer screening or sponsoring health-related contests at high schools. The director oversees these efforts, helping to plan programs and events, drawing up and managing the department budget, applying for funding, making long-range plans, and collaborating with the leaders of other departments and outside organizations. Bringing community groups together, guiding and assisting with their efforts, and providing information and resources they need can be a significant part of this job.

This is an office job, but one with a lot of interaction with community organizations and outside agencies. The director may be expected to represent the department at events that occur in the evenings and on weekends.

Education and Certification

At some local minority health offices, the director is a physician. At others, the director has an MPH, a master's degree in another related field, or a bachelor's degree with experience in local community health programs.

Core Competencies and Skills

- Ability to interact with and gain the trust of people from many different backgrounds
- Ability to handle multiple projects at once
- Understanding of epidemiologic principles
- Awareness of health equity issues and of existing programs to address health disparities
- Experience planning different types of outreach programs and knowledge of how to evaluate their success
- Experience with local minority groups and with the community organizations that are working to address their needs

Compensation

Salaries for local minority health directors reflect their qualifications as well as local budgets. In one region, typical salaries are in the range of $40,000 to $50,000; in another, a county director earns about $65,000. In a county where the director is a physician, the salary is closer to $150,000.

Workplaces

Minority health offices are found in health departments at every level of government. There is even a national Office of Minority Health.

Employment Outlook

There are not a lot of local-level offices of minority health yet, but this is a growing field. Meanwhile, people interested in minority health can also find positions elsewhere in local health departments, at state offices of minority health, or with nonprofit organizations.

For Further Information

■ Office of Minority Health, U.S. Department of Health and Human Services (OMH)
www.omhrc.gov

PUBLIC HEALTH PROFILE: Director, Office of Minority Health
Duane Herron, MPH
Minority Health Program Coordinator
Toledo-Lucas County Health Department, Toledo, OH

Describe the sort of work you do.

I work for the combined city and county health department, and I'm primarily assigned to a coalition of community groups that address health disparities through a number of different activities. I'm sort of a mediator, coordinating the activities within the coalition, supporting the work of the different groups, and helping them work together. The four major goals of my office are to report and monitor the health status of minority populations; to inform, educate, and empower our communities; to mobilize community partnerships; and to support policies and programs that focus on minority health initiatives.

What is a typical day like at your job?

Here's one recent day. I started in the office, spending a couple of hours writing and editing a strategic plan for the Office of Minority Health. Then I attended a conference on obesity. That meeting brought together local nonprofits, health care organizations, local government agencies, schools, and individuals from the community. Next, I had a lunch meeting with my program evaluator. We're working on a grant proposal for a youth development program, and we'll be replicating a program that another organization uses. Afterward I met with some of that organization's key staff members. I spent the rest of the day compiling what I learned and getting it back to the program evaluator.

Other tasks include looking at research data to learn where the most serious disparities are or to find other information we can use. I plan monthly coalition meetings with various community groups.

Continued

Sometimes an organization wants me to contribute an article or a column to their Web site, and I'm also responsible for our own Web site. I serve as a resource for various grant-funded programs in our area, too. Someone may be writing a grant proposal and want my advice.

What education or training do you have? Is it typical for your job?

My undergraduate degree is in community health, and my MPH focuses on health promotion and education. Not all the minority health program coordinators in Ohio have MPHs, but I think it's pretty common for a job like this.

What path did you take to get to the job you are in today?

I was working as a waiter when I decided to volunteer for an HIV prevention program. A year later, I was hired as that organization's HIV risk reduction specialist. My boss encouraged me to get a degree, and so I went to school to study community health. By the time I finished, I realized that I wanted to have an important influence, and the best way to start down that path seemed to be an MPH. My internship for the MPH was at the health department here, and I was assigned primarily to the local commission on minority health. I had a job as a health coach after graduation, but my supervisor at the health department knew I was interested in the coordinator job. When they needed to fill the position, they asked me to join their team.

Where might you go from here, if you wanted to advance your career?

Eventually, I'd like to go back to school for a PhD in public health epidemiology. I'm not sure whether I'll end up working in minority health or health disparities, specifically, but I'd like to have an upper-level job influencing health policy at the state or national level.

What is the worst or most challenging part of your job?

There are so many programs, and so many organizations trying to help, but the rate of disease is still rising. Because this is a relatively

Continued

new field, we don't always know yet what works best. I'm trying to help the community think critically about that, so we can work toward having effective programs that are driven by outcomes and will really make a difference.

What is the best part?

I like not knowing what's going to come next. Minority health is an emerging field, there is a lot of money available right now, and the field is growing. We have lots of opportunities for funding to continue addressing health disparities, and many states are looking to us for direction. I also enjoy the fact that I'm working on behalf of the community—and the people that I serve really do appreciate it.

What advice do you have for someone who is interested in your career?

Never underestimate the value of volunteer experiences. I understand community issues better because I was a volunteer in a community organization. After I got my degree, that experience also made it easier for me to find a job. Have a blend of academic experience, too, but also be able to apply it. When I was studying, I worried less about my GPA than about learning what I needed to do a good job.

PATIENT NAVIGATOR

Job Description

Some public health programs use "patient navigators" or "health navigators" to help patients find their way through the health care system. One important goal is to help make cancer screening programs more useful, by connecting members of underserved populations with timely medical care when a screening turns up a positive result. The role of a navigator stems from the fact that our health care system can be pretty confusing and intimidating. Big hospitals can seem like mazes. Dealing with bills and insurance can be frustrating and frightening. It can be especially hard for people who don't have good insurance, who aren't fluent in English, who don't fully understand how the health system works, or who come from communities that tend to think about health in ways doctors don't seem to "get." Navigators help patients set up the right appointments, find transportation, communicate with physicians (in English or otherwise), learn about their illnesses, and get answers to questions about insurance and costs. Some navigators even guide patients from the medical center entrance to the doctor's office. Navigators are also employed in public health research to guide patients through studies. There are navigators working with patients who require cancer care, refugees, people with HIV, and low-income patients.

Education and Certification

The required education depends on the program's design and on what services the navigator will provide. Some navigators don't need any special education at all. Some programs look for a bachelor's degree in a field related to health or experience as a community health worker. Some look for social workers or nurses.

Core Competencies and Skills

- Compassion
- Patience
- Good teaching skills
- Understanding of the different ways people react to stress and illness
- Ability to remain calm under stress
- Ability to judge the seriousness of situations and to prioritize needs
- Knowledge of how the health care system works, with at least basic understanding of medical terms

Compensation

Patient navigator salaries are related to the skills and knowledge required. They tend to be comparable to salaries for community health workers, nurses, or social workers, depending on the specific requirements.

Workplaces

Patient navigators work at universities, health departments, medical centers, and nonprofits.

Employment Outlook

The use of navigators is a developing field, and their role is still being studied. These jobs sometimes overlap with those of community health workers, social workers, or public health nurses. The outlook for these careers will probably become clearer over the next several years.

For Further Information

Patient navigators don't have a national organization as of this writing. For more information about patient navigation, visit:

■ National Cancer Institute (NCI)—Patient Navigation Research Program (PNRP)
  crchd.cancer.gov/pnp/pnrp-index.html

CORRECTIONAL MEDICINE PHYSICIAN

Job Description

A correctional medicine physician works within the city, county, state, or federal correctional system. These doctors provide clinical care for prisoners, and many also take part in designing and overseeing programs to protect the prisoners' health. Correctional medicine physicians may help to screen patients when they come into a facility, both to check for chronic illnesses like diabetes and to identify contagious diseases. Their work may include quality improvement efforts, working on changes that will help prevent medical problems, increase efficiency, and raise the standard of care. They may oversee disease control efforts, plan educational programs for inmates, help to write system-wide policies for the isolation and treatment of patients with certain infections, participate in disaster preparedness planning, or work in other ways to prevent illness and the spread of disease. They must adjust to changing population profiles, such as an increase in older patients with dementia. Rather than simply deal with problems as they occur in individual patients, a good prison health program incorporates surveillance, investigation of health problems, policy development, and evaluation—all elements of public health practice. These jobs tend to have predictable hours, with a limited number of nights and weekends on call. Physicians may be assigned to just one facility or may see patients at multiple locations.

Education and Certification

Correctional medicine physicians are usually trained in family practice or internal medicine. They must be able to handle a wide range of medical problems. Special certification is generally not required, but a certified Correctional Health Professional credential is available from the National Commission on Correctional Health Care.

Core Competencies and Skills

- Interest in handling complex cases
- Willingness to work with difficult people
- Broad knowledge of general medicine
- Understanding of the mental health issues common in correctional settings
- Tough skin and the ability to recognize and avoid attempts at manipulation
- Comfort with the atmosphere of a correctional facility, including locked doors and the presence of guards

Compensation

Salaries vary according to location, demand, local budgets, and responsibilities, and may or may not be comparable to typical physician salaries. In general, most internal medicine physicians earn at least $92,000, and the median salary is above $166,000. The median salary for family practice doctors and general practitioners is $157,000. Facility and system medical directors can earn higher salaries than physicians with less responsibility.

Workplaces

Correctional medicine physicians work at local jails and at state and federal prisons. Some states and local jurisdictions hire their own physicians. Others contract with private companies that hire physicians and assign them to sites.

Employment Outlook

Advertisements for correctional medicine physicians appear regularly. Increasingly, correctional systems are turning to outside corporations for medical staff, and many of these jobs are with such companies. However, the style of the work and the expectations may be different in these jobs, with less of a public health focus.

For Further Information

■ National Commission on Correctional Health Care (NCCHC)
www.ncchc.org
■ Society of Correctional Physicians (SCP)
www.corrdocs.org

PUBLIC HEALTH PROFILE: Correctional Medicine Physician
Elizabeth Sazie, MD, MPH, CCHP
Chief Medical Officer
Coffee Creek Correctional Facility
Oregon Department of Corrections, Wilsonville, OR

Describe the sort of work you do.

Coffee Creek Correctional Facility is the Oregon Department of Correction's intake center for all male and female inmates sentenced to over 1 year, and it is also the women's prison. (Men move to a male facility after the intake process.) Inmates can receive off-site medical care when needed, but we provide most of the care here on-site.

As chief medical officer, my top responsibility is to ensure that we offer high-quality care. In addition to my own clinical work, I provide leadership and staff development, do evaluation and supervision of the clinical staff, and help develop protocols and guidelines. I participate in continuous quality improvement, which includes making sure we are following protocols and examining statistics on deaths, adverse events, and hospitalizations. Another of my roles is overseeing the TB program for the state correctional system.

Continued

What is a typical day like at your job?

I usually come in and check my email, and then I go to the infirmary and make my rounds. The patients there are people who don't need to be in the hospital but do need extra care. They might be on oxygen or IVs, be recovering from surgery, or have something contagious so they can't be among the general population.

At noon, I call in to a state-wide conference call for an update about patients who are in the hospital. In the afternoon I handle certain special cases and consultations. I'm interested in HIV, so I do most of our HIV care. If I have patients going off-site for subspecialty care, I may need to call the consultants to coordinate care.

I fit my other work in around these responsibilities, including answering questions for the TB program and doing quality improvement. The past few days I've been going through charts to see who is receiving opiates, how often and why, and who is prescribing them. The nurses noticed that an increased number of patients were receiving these medications. I'm looking to see if there's a problem in our system and if so, what we need to do to address it.

What education or training do you have? Is it typical for your job?

I'm a licensed physician, which is essential for this job. Ideally, someone in this role should have a background in general medicine, either family practice or internal medicine.

What path did you take to get to the job you are in today?

After my internal medicine residency, my first job was at a university student health center. While I was there, we had an outbreak of Campylobacter. I worked with the health department and the CDC, and it was through that experience that I got connected to public health in the county. I took a part-time job as county health officer, investigating foodborne outbreaks and communicable disease cases and serving as medical director of the jail. I earned my MPH during that time. When the health department downsized, there weren't a lot of other opportunities in our area for public health doctors, so I

Continued

practiced with an internal medicine group. But at a local forum on criminality, I happened to meet an administrator of the Department of Corrections Health Services. She asked me, "Why don't you come work with us?" I said, "But you guys don't do public health." And she said, "Yes we do!"

Where might you go from here, if you wanted to advance your career?

The only way to advance in this department would be if my director left—and I really like him, so I want him to stay. I suppose if I wanted to I could work for a private corporation that provides health care in prisons. Or I could do clinical medicine somewhere else.

What is the worst or most challenging part of your job?

The way things work in government can be really inefficient. At one point we had a temporary assistant we really wanted to hire permanently, but there wasn't a job category that she officially fit into. And so we couldn't hire her.

What is the best part?

Back at the health department, I was the only MD doing that kind of work, and even within the state there weren't a lot of us. I felt isolated. Here, my staff and I bounce cases off each other, and we help each other out. It makes it fun. Also, I take care of patients with very complex problems—both physical and mental—and it is just fascinating. I like figuring out how to help them.

What advice do you have for someone who is interested in your career?

We like to hire people who are experienced and who are non-judgmental. We have a lot of patients who are very practiced at manipulating people, and you have to be able to differentiate between the real problem and the secondary gain. If we had a real newbie in here, I think he or she would be at risk of being taken advantage of.

DISEASE PREVENTION ACTIVIST

Job Description

This isn't necessarily a job title you'll find in the help wanted ads, although it does sometimes turn up. It describes a range of opportunities to work for improvements in disease prevention and health promotion. Many of these activists are working to reduce health disparities and raise the overall health of certain minority groups. These people are the heart of upstart community health organizations and small foundations that focus on preventing breast cancer or heart disease or birth defects or AIDS. They give presentations at town council meetings, put together community events, devise creative ways to encourage behavior change, raise money for programs, and inform the media about overlooked populations or hidden dangers. These activists help keep health issues in the public eye, pick up the slack where health agencies are not meeting needs, and encourage public policy that will support a healthier society.

Their day-to-day work varies, but it can include gathering signatures, writing grant proposals, sending out press releases, and organizing public events. Activists may also work directly with groups and individual patients to provide health or nutrition education, encourage safe behaviors, hand out supplies such as condoms or clean needles, or do screening tests. As an organization grows or an activist's career advances, these same people may find themselves running organizations, advising health officials, and overseeing large health promotion campaigns.

Education and Certification

Just about anyone, at any level of education, can take a stand to promote public health. Commitment to the cause is the most important qualification. Jobs with activist organizations may require specific skills or knowledge: a public relations person to raise the organization's profile in the press, a community organizer to pull together broad support for a ban on smoking in restaurants.

Core Competencies and Skills

- Creative thinking
- Belief that change is possible

- Stubbornness about accomplishing goals, plus flexibility about how to reach them
- Knack for persuasion
- Excellent communication skills
- Initiative and the ability to see projects through to the end, in spite of obstacles
- Knowledge of the medical, social, and cultural issues surrounding disease prevention

Compensation

People who do this type of work often feel that personal satisfaction is the most important reward. Then again, this work can lead to increasing responsibility and respect, and it can be a steppingstone to other opportunities. Compensation varies greatly according to funding, responsibility, and the size of the organization.

Workplaces

Activists generally work for nonprofit organizations. These can be small, local organizations—or groups that started out small and have since grown to have a national reach.

Employment Outlook

Finding paid work as a disease prevention activist can be somewhat challenging, because organizations often have limited funding and there are many young people who are interested in starting out in this type of work. Employee turnover and the ongoing need for improvements in public health make it likely that jobs will continue to be available, but it may take patience and persistence to find one.

For Further Information

- There is no single organization for activists involved in disease prevention. Instead, explore the Web sites of local and national advocacy organizations that focus on a particular health topic and/or population. Also see the Web sites of local minority health coalitions.

PRESIDENT AND CEO, AREA AGENCY ON AGING

Job Description

Area agencies on aging (AAAs) are regional nonprofit organizations designated by state governments to address the needs of older adults. These agencies are concerned with issues such as eliminating physical and emotional abuse of elderly people, making sure that homebound elders have nutritious food to eat, and connecting eligible people to social services. There are programs to help elders "age in place," which means staying in their own houses and apartments instead of nursing homes. Many sponsor community centers where older adults can socialize, exercise, and take classes, or "day care" centers for people who need a safe place to go while their caregivers work. AAAs often do not provide direct services, but instead contract with local service providers who carry out the day-to-day work of the programs.

The chief executive officer (CEO) of an AAA guides the agency's work. This includes setting short- and long-term priorities, ensuring that programs conform to federal and local regulations, and helping the agency adapt if local needs change. The CEO is responsible for ensuring that funding is available and that contracts with service providers are appropriate. The CEO has administrative duties such as overseeing the budget (with the help of a financial officer), hiring and supervising certain personnel, interacting with elected officials to advocate for seniors, and meeting with leaders of other organizations and agencies to collaborate on service and policy efforts and to make sure that goals are aligned.

Education and Certification

These executives generally have at least a bachelor's degree, and some have higher degrees; there are MPAs, social workers, lawyers, and others. Most have prior experience as administrators of services related to aging or as administrators or supervisors in other public programs.

Core Competencies and Skills

- Excellent management skills, for both personnel and finance
- Strong verbal and written communication skills

- Knack for political and community networking and an understanding of public relations
- Awareness of the issues faced by elder adults in general, and of issues specific to the local population
- Understanding of government funding processes and knowledge of how to obtain funding
- Understanding of laws, regulations, and services related to elder affairs
- Understanding of epidemiologic principles and program evaluation techniques

Compensation

Based on tax forms filed by AAAs in recent years, salaries are often in the range of $80,000 to $120,000.

Workplaces

Most states have multiple AAAs, and several have 10 or more. Some AAAs are incorporated into nonprofits that cover other social services, as well; in these cases, the person in charge of the aging component often has the title of Director. A few states do not have AAAs; instead, programs are administered through a central government office.

Employment Outlook

The prospects for this specific job are limited by the number of AAAs. For those who are interested in administering services to promote the health of older adults, there are additional opportunities within nonprofit organizations and at government offices on aging.

For Further Information

- National Association of Area Agencies on Aging (n4a)
  www.n4a.org
- American Society on Aging (ASA)
  www.asaging.org

■ National Association of State Units on Aging (NASUA)
www.nasua.org
■ American Public Health Association—Gerontological Health section
www.apha.org/membergroups/sections/aphasections/gh

REFERENCE

U.S. Department of Health and Human Services, Office of Minority Health. (October 21, 2009). *Data/Statistics: African American profile, American Indian/Alaska Native profile,* and *Hispanic/Latino profile.* Retrieved from http://minorityhealth.hhs.gov/templates/browse.aspx?lvl=1&lvlID=2

16 Mental Health

The World Health Organization (WHO) defines health as "a state of complete physical, mental, and social well-being and not merely the absence of disease or infirmity." People who are mentally healthy are best able to cope with life's stresses, do productive work, realize their own potential, and contribute to their communities.

Mental illness is not rare. It has been estimated that 46% of U.S. adults will experience an anxiety disorder, an impulse-control disorder, a substance abuse disorder, or a mood disorder like depression at some point in their lives. A few years ago, the financial cost of mental illness in the United States was estimated at $150 billion each year. And yet, the majority of people who have been diagnosed with mental illness are not receiving treatment. There are also important differences in mental health outcomes among various socioeconomic, racial, and ethnic groups.

Public health professionals are addressing mental health in several ways. They are exploring patterns of illness and looking for risk factors that could lead to targeted interventions or new methods for prevention. They are working to increase awareness of mental health problems and reduce the stigma associated with them. They are seeking ways to improve the efficiency and effectiveness of our mental health system. And they are creating many different types of programs that address mental health needs at the community, state, and national levels.

This chapter is relatively short, for two reasons. First, other types of public health efforts sometimes incorporate mental health issues. And second, mental health and public health have, historically, been treated as separate fields. In recent years, there has been increasing interest in integrating mental health and public health, and the future may bring new efforts and new career opportunities.

Other jobs that may involve work related to mental health include medical officer, public health nurse, health educator, health promotion coordinator, helpline advisor, behavioral scientist, injury prevention specialist, corporate medical director, disease prevention activist, program officer, medical director, and the careers in the chapter on maternal and child health.

MENTAL HEALTH RESEARCHER

Job Description

Researchers in mental health study the causes and effects of mental illness and hunt for new ways to treat and manage psychiatric disorders. In the public health realm, this includes population-level issues such as how neighborhood characteristics influence mental health, how a disaster might trigger psychiatric problems, why people in certain groups might be more likely to develop mental illnesses, or how the health care system can do a better job of helping people who are mentally ill. Mental health researchers often work in partnership with other researchers and clinical staff. They raise funds for their projects by applying for grants from the government, nonprofit organizations, or industry.

Projects might include examining national data to look for trends in the use of mental health care, gathering information from community members to find out what people with similar mental health problems have in common, or trying to find the best way to provide mental health services. Researchers share what they have learned through conference presentations and journal articles. Some mental health researchers use the results of their studies to help design and implement public health programs. A mental health researcher might also speak to the media or offer advice to policymakers. This can be primarily a desk job, or it can involve going out into the community, conducting focus groups, and interviewing patients. Experienced researchers often have assistants carry out the day-to-day research tasks while they focus on designing studies, raising funds, and analyzing and presenting results.

Education and Certification

Most public health scientists who specialize in mental health have advanced degrees, usually PhDs, in fields such as clinical psychology, sociology, social work, or other related subjects. Some have alternative degrees at the doctoral level, such as Doctor of Science (DSc) or DrPH, and some are doctors or nurses. It is possible to become a researcher in mental health with just an MPH, but as a general rule, a doctoral level degree will allow access to more prestigious jobs. Many researchers are also university professors, and this title requires a doctoral-level degree.

Core Competencies and Skills

- Curiosity
- Initiative
- Persistence
- Appreciation for cultural and socioeconomic diversity
- Strong writing skills
- Training in study design, epidemiology, and statistics
- Ability to work independently and also to work with a team
- Knowledge of or experience in the clinical side of mental health treatment

Compensation

Salaries depend on type of employer, background, and responsibilities. As an example, psychology professors in doctoral departments earned from about $50,000 to about $150,000, depending on rank and experience, during the 2008 to 2009 academic year. Mental health researchers who work for private firms tend to earn more, at the same level of experience, than those at academic institutions.

Workplaces

Researchers in the field of mental health often work at universities, where they may also teach classes, and at government agencies and nonprofit organizations. There are also opportunities at private consulting firms, where researchers do work requested by government agencies or other organizations.

Employment Outlook

The outlook depends on the availability of funding, since much of this type of research depends on government grants. Funding may be somewhat easier to find now than it was several years ago; future jobs will depend on the level of interest in preventing and treating mental health problems. Being creative about proposed research—looking for ways to connect ideas with government interests—can be helpful when looking for a job or applying for grants.

For Further Information

- American Public Health Association—Mental Health Section
  www.apha.org/membergroups/sections/aphasections/mental
- Substance Abuse and Mental Health Services Administration (SAMHSA)
  www.samhsa.gov
- National Institute of Mental Health (NIMH)
  www.nimh.nih.gov

PUBLIC HEALTH PROFILE: Mental Health Researcher
Leigh Ann Simmons, PhD, MFT
Assistant Professor of Medicine
Duke University School of Medicine, Durham, NC

Describe the sort of work you do.

I'm based at Duke University's Center for Research on Prospective Health Care. There are two aspects to my work. One is trying to understand the contributors to mental health. I study biological factors, psychological factors, social factors, and even environmental factors—everything from how your brain works to where you live. Then I take that information and develop interventions. One example is a program called Blue to You. My colleague and I conducted a survey about depression and then used the results to create tailored educational modules for youth group meetings, senior centers, churches, and other community settings. Another project I'm

Continued

working on is developing a parenting education and mindfulness intervention for mothers with depression. The goal is to improve mom's mental health and reduce the risk of problems for the child.

What is a typical day like at your job?

I don't have a typical day, and that's what makes it fun. There are several elements in a typical week. One is sitting with my team members, hashing out research ideas and brainstorming about papers or grant proposals to write. Another is reading. To inform my work, I look up other people's research papers and read their findings. I spend about 50% of my time writing, creating grant applications, research papers, and institutional review board (IRB) proposals. The IRB is the ethics committee at the university, and all research projects require their approval.

I'm personally involved in the design and implementation of all my research projects. Once a study is up and running, my research assistants often handle the day-to-day work, and I check in with them to see how things are going. I train them to recruit patients, explain the study, and collect information, and I'll sit with them the first few times to ensure they understand what to do.

My research assistants are usually undergraduate and graduate students, and I serve as a mentor to them. I also have conference calls and email correspondence about multicenter studies I'm involved in.

What education or training do you have? Is it typical for your job?

My job requires a doctoral-level degree. In addition to my PhD in Child and Family Development, I have a Master of Family Therapy (MFT) degree. At the University of Kentucky, where I had my first academic job, I learned more about women's health and clinical research through a faculty training program.

What path did you take to get to the job you are in today?

I had originally thought I would go to medical school, so after college I worked at an adolescent medicine practice. I really liked talking with the patients about their lives, but I wasn't as interested in

Continued

clinical practice. I worked in medical publishing for a while, and then decided to go back to school and earn the MFT. During my master's program, I got a job as a research coordinator, and I just loved it. That's what led me to earn a PhD. My dissertation focused on the relationship between poverty and health in rural, low-income mothers. While doing this study, I noticed that a huge number of these women were suffering from depression, far more than the national average. I found that really interesting, and I wanted to learn more about why that was and what I could do about it.

Where might you go from here, if you wanted to advance your career?

At an academic center, rising through the ranks to full professor is one possible goal. Many universities have centers that focus on mental health research and policy, so directing a center, at some point in my career, is also a possibility. I could even start my own research center someday, if I get really ambitious.

What is the worst or most challenging part of your job?

There can be an ivory tower phenomenon. People are working on their own research in isolation. I try to keep that from happening in my own work, but you can end up working with the same group of people most of the time and not knowing what is going on in another department.

What is the best part?

I love collaborating with people. I love the synergy of getting into a room of people with different perspectives, and working together to come up with a really great research idea. If I could just come up with ideas all the time, I would be thrilled!

What advice do you have for someone who is interested in your career?

I believe I'm doing something for the larger good, and I think that belief has helped me be successful. Sitting around reading research articles

Continued

won't be any fun if its not something you are really interested in. It is being interested, and caring, and wanting to make a difference that gets me through the harder days. Whenever you consider participating in research, think: "Is this aligned with who I really want to be?"

PUBLIC HEALTH SOCIAL WORKER

Job Description

Social workers help people use the resources available to them to cope with physical and mental illness, as well as other challenges they face in their lives. They connect people with available services, provide counseling and guidance, and look for ways to maximize functioning and minimize disability. Public health social workers are trained to use epidemiologic methods and research evidence to identify psychosocial challenges and find solutions at the population level. They can use this training in many different ways. They can be involved in creating and running city, county, or state social work programs, shaping public policy, tracking social and mental health problems, and finding new or better ways to address these issues. A public health social worker might provide guidance for domestic violence prevention programs, helping the planners understand the personal issues that community members face. He or she might identify an emerging trend of substance abuse in a neighborhood and devise a way to intervene. Or, he or she might help evaluate social work efforts to see if they are making a difference.

Some public health social workers provide direct service at community clinics or through health department programs, as part of systematic efforts to address problems in specific populations. Typical roles include helping adults and their families find services and develop coping skills to reduce the risk of elder abuse, assisting teenage mothers as they learn to become good parents, helping refugees overcome past trauma and new challenges, and helping HIV/AIDS patients deal with the illness so they can continue working, avoid complications, and reduce the risk of transmitting the infection to others.

Education and Certification

A bachelor's degree in social work is enough for some entry-level jobs (and some employers will accept a bachelor's degree in a related field such as psychology). However, social workers with Master of Social Work (MSW) degrees will find more opportunities in public health, particularly if they have pursued training in community-level work. Several schools of social work offer combined MSW/MPH degrees. Licensing requirements vary by state, but in general a social worker must have a license to do clinical practice.

Core Competencies and Skills

- Empathy
- Patience and willingness to appreciate slow or incremental change
- Good listening and communication skills
- Strong problem-solving skills and the ability to think on your feet
- Ability to assess needs on a community level, and to use epidemiologic principles and research evidence to design and evaluate interventions
- Ability to work with people from different backgrounds, and to encourage consensus among people with different interests and needs
- Knowledge of local, state, and federal programs that provide assistance to people in need

Compensation

For most social workers with MSW degrees, a salary in the range of $40,000 to $60,000 is typical. Salaries tend to be lower for those with only bachelor's degrees. Social workers in high-level supervisory or leadership positions can earn $100,000 per year or more.

Workplaces

Public health social workers are found at state, city, county health departments, and at federal agencies dedicated to serving the country's physical and mental health needs. They also work at nonprofit organizations, on both the local and national levels.

Employment Outlook

The number of job openings and the number of social workers looking for work are expected to be in rough balance over the next several years.

Several states report a shortage of public health social workers or expect to see a shortage soon. At the same time, public health social workers do often find that their special combination of skills is not fully recognized, and so finding work that makes use of both clinical knowledge and public health skills can require a bit of creativity.

For Further Information

- American Public Health Association—Social Work Section
  www.apha.org/membergroups/sections/aphasections/socialwork
- Association of State and Territorial Public Health Social Workers (ASTPHSW)
  astphsw.org
- National Association of Social Workers (NASW)
  www.naswdc.org

PUBLIC HEALTH PROFILE: Public Health Social Worker
Mamie Elmore, LMSW
Social Work Director, Region 4
South Carolina Department of Health and Environmental Control (DHEC), Florence, SC

Describe the sort of work you do.

My title is Director of Social Work for a 10-county region in rural South Carolina. I monitor and facilitate professional social work practice for the region, provide direct services, assist with personnel issues and staffing assignments, provide guidance to staff as they do their work, and ensure they receive up-to-date training. The counties here have limited resources. Our social workers address the psychosocial issues and/or barriers that prohibit individuals from reaching their optimal status, and assist citizens to effectively utilize available resources.

We provide social work services to patients in the following program areas: Home Health, HIV/AIDS, Baby Net, Breast and Cervical Cancer, Maternal and Child Health, Family Planning, and Tuberculosis. Presently, I am working with a collaborative network of diverse stakeholders to recruit and educate leaders on how to manage arthritis and to develop a network of leaders to promote the message in the local community.

Continued

What is a typical day like at your job?

A typical day is fragmented, with numerous interruptions. The primary focus of my work is the Arthritis Foundation Initiative. I schedule events and assure that the leaders are qualified to teach assigned classes. In the midst of a scheduled assignment, such as ordering supplies for a class, I might receive a telephone call concerning a referral or an ethical issue that requires immediate attention. I may get a call that an HIV client has presented for "walk-in" services and there is no social worker available, so I have to stop and assess the client's needs. Upon return to my office my supervisor may call for an administrative report that is needed to meet an unscheduled deadline. The Arthritis Foundation DHEC State Director may call and need immediate information. I may receive a call from a client who has been newly diagnosed with breast cancer and does not know how she can pay her hospital bill. A social worker from another county may call, needing consultation in working through a difficult situation with a client. The day is gone and the initial project I started on is still pending.

What education or training do you have? Is it typical for your job?

My educational background is standard for a public health social worker. I have a bachelor's degree in sociology and a Master of Social Work degree.

What path did you take to get to the job you are in today?

Between the bachelor's and the master's I was a Tuberculosis Disease Investigator with the New York City Department of Health. After graduate school, I worked for a nonprofit organization, monitoring home day care centers to assure they were compliant with standards of operation. I observed that the day care providers were overwhelmed with the issues that children and their families were facing—child abuse, drug addiction, and domestic violence. The organization obtained funding for preventive services, and I was instrumental in

Continued

setting up that program. Upon relocating to South Carolina, I was employed as a Home Health Social Worker with DHEC. I have since worked in all program areas (children with developmental delays, HIV, family planning, maternal and child health, environmental quality control, tuberculosis, arthritis, and chronic disease, etc.). Then I was selected as Director of Social Work.

Where might you go from here, if you wanted to advance your career?

For someone who desires to move up the career ladder, the next step would be a state program director or consultant position. The Office of Public Health Social Work career ladder consists of direct practice social workers, Region Social Work Directors, State Program Consultants and a State Office of Public Heath Social Work Director. Research and epidemiology are areas social workers need to explore, as we have so much insight and pertinent information that can affect societal change.

What is the worst or most challenging part of your job?

Our region ranks close to the top in the state for health disparities, unemployment, and illiteracy. With the high health disparity, limited resources and nine master social workers to cover 10 counties, we are stretched and pulled in numerous directions. Issues, concerns, and needs are identified but we have limited staff to address or promote policy change or policy development. Given these challenges, the staff is not able to be a true change agent.

What is the best part?

The best parts are working with people who care about their community and want to make a change; promoting communication strategies that are responsive to community issues, priorities, and solutions; and engaging a broad range of stakeholders in prevention and intervention strategies to promote optimal health.

I love being able to tell someone, "You can get through this. You have power hidden within you that you have not used." This is the mission for which I awake every day of my life.

Continued

What advice do you have for someone who is interested in your career?

I would first ask, is the field of social work a true interest? One should not become a social worker just because of a desire to help people, as you can do that in many other ways. To me, this is a calling. It is very rewarding, yet emotionally challenging. One should search their heart for their true calling. Make sure you are ready to work in communities with limited to no resources and to help people who do not yet know their innate abilities or are afraid to take a risk. As a public health social worker you will be on the front lines every day, fighting and advocating for those disenfranchised citizens who need your expertise and skill.

COORDINATOR, BEHAVIORAL HEALTH PROGRAM

Job Description

There are behavioral health programs that address certain mental and behavioral health issues on a population or community level. For example, there are community-based efforts to reduce methamphetamine abuse. Colleges often have campaigns to convince students that binge drinking is dangerous. There are programs to destigmatize depression and other forms of mental illness, so that sufferers will seek help. The people who run these programs assess community needs, examine past efforts, and determine, based on the best evidence, what is most likely to help. They may have hands-on roles, such as leading classes or visiting community members, or they may be primarily office-based—coordinating the health educators, nurses, substance abuse counselors, and other experts who go out into the field. Applying for funding and managing the budget is part of the job, as well.

Education and Certification

Requirements depend on the needs of the specific program. Some managers or coordinators of these programs are social workers, some are trained as substance abuse counselors or as health educators, some have master's degrees in public health or public administration. There is an optional Certified Prevention Specialist certification for people doing drug and alcohol abuse prevention work, requiring a certain amount of education and experience and an examination.

Core Competencies and Skills

- Creativity
- Good management skills
- Ability to handle multiple responsibilities at once
- Knowledge of how to assess community needs
- Understanding of issues in mental and behavioral health
- Ability to locate and understand research evidence for behavioral health programs
- Understanding of the population being targeted
- Knowledge of how to implement and evaluate programs

Compensation

There are no national statistics for this type of job, but salaries tend to be relatively modest. A typical example is the range of $35,000 to $58,000 for a substance abuse prevention coordinator on one university campus. A program coordinator at a small county health department or nonprofit might have a salary in the $30,000 range; someone who manages multiple programs for a larger county might earn $80,000.

Workplaces

There are behavioral health programs based at local health departments, human services offices, public school districts, and colleges and universities. Some are run by nonprofit organizations or for-profit companies. There are also programs at tribal organizations and in the military.

Employment Outlook

Funding for these types of programs has been stable in recent years. There is significant employee turnover, due in part to the relatively low salaries. The future of these types of programs will depend on government funding and on interest among the public health community.

For Further Information

See the links in the mental health researcher description. Also of interest are:

- National Association of State Alcohol/Drug Abuse Directors (NASADAD) *www.nasadad.org*
- National Association of County Behavioral Health and Developmental Disability Directors (NACBHDD) *www.nacbhdd.org*

HOMELESS SERVICES EDUCATOR

Job Description

A homeless services educator (or someone with a similar title) teaches doctors, nurses, other health care workers, and other service providers how to work with homeless clients. Many homeless people are mentally ill, and they have trouble cooperating with doctors or following instructions for their health. Others are simply dealing with the incredible stress of having no permanent place to shower, sleep, and eat. Homeless patients may have trouble obtaining medication or getting back to the doctor's office for follow-up appointments. Unfortunately, our health care system isn't set up to address those challenges. Further, many health care providers and public health program personnel do not understand the special issues that homeless people face or know how to accommodate them.

To address this system-level problem, organizations that specialize in helping the homelessness have begun to offer trainings for staff at medical settings, homeless shelters, drug and alcohol treatment centers, dedicated homeless health care programs, and other places where homeless people seek help. Trainers address issues such as constructive communication, hospital discharge planning, and local services available to the homeless. They may cover techniques for dealing with difficult people, motivational interviewing, the emotional effects of violence, and the mental illnesses and infectious diseases that are particularly common among the homeless. A trainer's job may include tasks such as creating educational materials and slide presentations, travelling to clinics and hospitals, and conducting classes. The job can also involve "training the trainers," teaching doctors, nurses, social workers, and others so that they can share the information with colleagues.

Education and Certification

Organizations that offer this type of training set their own individual requirements. One potentially appropriate background would be a degree in health education.

Core Competencies and Skills

- Good communication skills
- Understanding of psychology
- Ability to recognize what specific groups of health care providers are likely to know and need to know, to create a lesson plan, and to convey needed information clearly and concisely
- Experience working with diverse homeless populations and knowledge of the challenges that homeless people face

Compensation

This job most closely resembles that of a health educator. In 2008, the median salary for health educators was $44,000, and most earned between $26,000 and $78,000.

Workplaces

People who do these types of trainings usually work at nonprofit organizations or at consulting firms.

Employment Outlook

There are not many people working full time as homeless services educators. More often, this type of work is part of a job incorporating other efforts to address the needs of homeless or other at-risk populations. Public health professionals who have the necessary knowledge could take the initiative to seek grant funding for a local program. Contacting an organization that already provides this type of education would be a good start.

For Further Information

- National Health Care for the Homeless Council (HCH)
  www.nhchc.org
- Homelessness Resource Center
  www.nrchmi.samhsa.gov

REFERENCES

Giles, W. H., & Collins, J. L. (2010). A shared worldview: Mental health and public health at the crossroads. *Preventing Chronic Disease, 7*(1). Retrieved from http://www.cdc.gov/pcd/issues/2010/jan/09_0181.htm

Satcher, D., & Druss, B. G. (2010). Bridging mental health and public health. *Preventing Chronic Disease, 7*(1). Retrieved from http://www.cdc.gov/pcd/issues/2010/jan/09_0133.htm

Williams, S. M., Chapman, D., & Lando J. (2005). *The role of public health in mental health promotion. Morbidity and Mortality Weekly Report, 54*(34), 841–842.

World Health Organization. (2007). Fact sheet 220. Mental health: Strengthening mental health promotion. Retrieved from http://www.who.int/mediacentre/factsheets/fs220/en. Accessed on March 23, 2010

17 Public Health Law, Regulations, and Policies

There is a difference between public health laws, regulations, and policies. Laws are enacted by legislators—by votes in Congress, state legislatures, or city councils. Regulations are the rules put in place by government agencies to carry out the laws. Policy is a more general term used variously to describe laws, regulations, and agencies' overall plans and strategies.

Another important clarification is the difference between "health law" and "public health law." A prominent public health lawyer, Lawrence Gostin, has defined public health law as referring to the government's powers and duties to "assure the conditions for people to be healthy." His definition also includes the limitations on these powers, which prevent the state from unduly restricting citizens' rights. Health law is a much broader category. Practitioners of health law include medical malpractice attorneys and lawyers who represent hospitals and insurance companies.

While nearly every public health professional's work interacts with laws and regulations in some way, the jobs in this chapter focus largely on the laws and regulations themselves.

ADVOCACY DIRECTOR

Job Description

The advocacy director is the connection between a public health organization and the political world. "Advocacy" is about encouraging government officials to support policy that favors the organization's goals. That means getting laws passed and getting line items in federal, state, and city budgets. It also means working to get services provided in a way the organization thinks will be most effective. To make these things happen, the advocacy director keeps up-to-date on the latest news and policy issues, gets to know politicians and their staff members, and encourages the public to call their representatives and show their support. The advocacy director plans events to raise awareness about public health issues and prepares reports summarizing current policy issues and needs. The advocacy director also maintains relationships with related foundations, companies, and agencies, so they can present a united front. The job often involves a combination of deskwork and meetings outside the office. It may also require travel. (This job can also be called "Policy Director," "Director of Government Relations," or another variation.)

Education and Certification

An advocacy director's background usually includes at least a bachelor's degree plus training or experience in politics and health care issues. A master's degree in a related field (such as public policy, nonprofit management, or the organization's health focus) makes a candidate more competitive and is required for some jobs.

Core Competencies and Skills

- Understanding of relevant health care issues
- Tact and a knack for persuasion
- Excellent written and verbal communication skills
- Personal interest in the organization's goals
- Knowledge of the legislative process
- Experience with advocacy or grassroots organizing

Compensation

Salary depends on the size of the organization and the scope of the job. National salary surveys suggest averages of about $68,000 to $76,000. At a tiny nonprofit, it could be as low as the $20,000s, while a high-level job at a large nonprofit could pay well above the average.

Workplaces

Advocacy directors usually work at nonprofit organizations. The job title also exists at for-profit businesses, but the work is generally geared toward increasing the company's opportunities for profit.

Employment Outlook

As a whole, jobs in advocacy, grantmaking, and civic organizations are expected to expand. Landing a job as advocacy director for a very specific cause or organization can be challenging; a good bet is to look for opportunities to gain experience in organizing or advocacy, and then work toward eventually obtaining a job in the desired area.

For Further Information

- National Council of Nonprofits
  www.councilofnonprofits.org
- Center for Lobbying in the Public Interest (CLPI)
  www.clpi.org

POLICY ANALYST

Job Description

A policy analyst keeps track of laws, regulations, and funding related to an organization's or agency's interests. This includes current policy, changes that are being discussed, and changes that might occur in the future. The policy analyst also tracks the impact of existing laws and policies, looks at current public health programs, and explores the potential effects of policy changes. To do this, he or she consults with outside experts, conducts research, and keeps up with news reports, government documents, and outside organizations' and agencies' efforts. Then, he or she prepares reports incorporating all this information. The reports may be used to argue for a certain policy change, or they may be intended to help with decision making. Policy analysts also share their knowledge with legislators, agency officials, and community stakeholders. A policy analyst job can incorporate elements of program evaluation, data analysis, and policy development, as well. Some policy analysts also create fact sheets, write editorials, speak to the media, or even appear on television. Policy analysts spend much of their time on the computer, researching the issues and writing reports; they also attend meetings on-and off-site and sometimes travel to program locations and conferences.

Education and Certification

A policy analyst generally needs at least a master's degree in public health, public policy, or another field related to public health policy issues. A bachelor's degree with strong experience in policy, such as a job as a legislative aide, will suffice for some positions. For some positions, a PhD, MD, or JD is most appropriate, and some policy analysts were originally trained as social workers or nurses. It is helpful to have at least some work experience that relates to the policy topic when applying for a first job as a policy analyst.

Core Competencies and Skills

- Excellent writing and presentation skills
- Knack for analytical and strategic thinking
- Ability to understand complex information and to summarize it in a logical way
- Ability to create working relationships with experts from outside agencies, organizations, and academic centers
- Knowledge of government and legislative processes and of how to find information related to laws and policies
- Additional knowledge relevant to the organization or agency's interests
- For some jobs, good negotiation skills to bring scientists, public health experts, and legislators together on policy plans

Compensation

There is no national summary of policy analysts' salaries. In federal government agencies, policy analysts who are very experienced can earn $100,000 per year or more; a typical starting salary would be in the range of $65,000 to $75,000. Certain well-funded nonprofits also offer generous pay to well-qualified analysts. For people who have little experience or who work on small projects or at small organizations, salaries can be as low as the $30,000s.

Workplaces

Policy analysts interested in public health usually work for nonprofits or government agencies. Some work for consulting firms or "think tanks" that specialize in interpreting policy issues.

Employment Outlook

It is difficult to assess the employment outlook, because policy analyst jobs can have various titles. Some have responsibilities that overlap with other jobs, such as program officer. However, since this job is essential to major organizations that seek to influence policy, it is likely that job openings will continue to be available. Looking for a lower-level job related to policy, where you can start to gain the required experience, is one way to get your foot in the door.

For Further Information

Policy analysts often belong to organizations that match their specific interests, including APHA. Here are some other related links:

- Health Affairs
  www.healthaffairs.org
- AcademyHealth
  www.academyhealth.org

PUBLIC HEALTH PROFILE: Policy Analyst
Jennifer Greaser, RN, MSN
Public Health Analyst
Centers for Disease Control and Prevention, Washington, DC

Describe the sort of work you do.

I work for CDC's Washington Office. The Office has two main functions. The first is analysis, analyzing legislation and other policies and their impact on public health. The second is communicating with

Continued

policymakers in Congress, at other federal agencies, and at the state and local levels, to provide the information they need when they are creating legislation that may affect public health. A good example is the work we've been doing for the Child Nutrition Reauthorization. We have been working with colleagues to provide the latest scientific evidence about nutrition, so that legislators can make the best decisions as they update child nutrition programs.

What is a typical day like at your job?

The work can be very fast-paced. Policymakers are under their own deadlines, and sometimes their staff will call and want an answer within an hour. At other times, I have days or weeks to do an analysis.

An analysis starts with reading the original legislation or policy and any related materials. I talk with CDC scientists and other researchers to learn about the science behind a policy and how a new decision could impact research. I speak with public health planners about potential effects on public health programs. Then I have to find out what happens in the day-to-day world. Say I'm looking a policy that aims to increase children's fruit and vegetable consumption by changing what's in school lunches. I'll talk to experts about issues such as what children are likely to eat, whether schools have enough refrigerators, and if their kitchens are equipped to steam vegetables.

At times, I go out to see the programs that would be affected or arrange for congressmen or staff members to do a site visit. Once I have the background information, I arrange conference calls or meetings with legislators and their staff members, and sometimes also with CDC scientists, and we'll talk through the issues. I help "translate" the science and summarize what I have learned. Sometimes I'm also asked to write policy papers for my Director or to provide a written review of legislation.

What education or training do you have? Is it typical for your job?

I have a BSN and a master's in nursing health policy, but people in this job tend to have MPHs, JDs, or MPAs. There are also some MDs and other RNs. With experience in a legislative office, a bachelor's degree can be enough.

Continued

What path did you take to get to the job you are in today?

I started out as a nurse doing clinical care. I got my master's degree while I was still working in the hospital, and then I was accepted into an HHS career development program called the Emerging Leaders Program (ELP). In the ELP, you start at a low- to mid-range job and do rotations to different agencies. You're promoted after each year, and at the end of 2 years you can be hired on full time. That's how I got started in my current job.

Where might you go from here, if you wanted to advance your career?

To round out my experience more, I might want to spend some time at another federal agency whose policies impact public health—such as the Department of Education or the Department of Transportation. When you're trying to influence policy through the public health lens, it is helpful to understand the lenses that other agencies are looking through. More generally, the next step for someone in my role might be to become director of legislative affairs for a nonprofit organization.

What is the worst or most challenging part of your job?

With policy, you can be working on something for years before you see the results. Policymaking involves a lot of steps, a lot of influences, and a lot of players. You really have to have patience to see it through. I also find that sitting at a desk all day long can be tough. Sometimes I just have to get up and take a walk.

What is the best part?

For me, the eye-opening moment was when I realized that there are so many things that impact public health, and so many things that policymakers haven't necessarily thought of. I like knowing that we provide really good quality science to legislators and that we are helping them make the best decisions. Working at the federal level is really exciting, too. I'm close to the action, working directly with the people who are making important decisions.

Continued

> ## What advice do you have for someone who is interested in your career?
>
> If you're interested this job and want to have a competitive edge, get experience in some kind of a policy office. That will also help you decide if this is the kind of work you want to do. If you can't get an internship in Congress, look for state or local opportunities or do a summer internship in the legislative affairs office at a nonprofit. If you're already out of school, look for fellowships and other government programs designed for people with your background.

HEALTH LEGISLATIVE ASSISTANT

Job Description

State legislators and members of Congress have a lot to keep track of—bills, constituents with concerns, lobbyists raising new issues. Legislative assistants help make it possible for legislators to do their work by serving as the in-office experts on vital issues. The health legislative assistant focuses specifically on health care matters including public health, does the background research on important issues, and helps the legislator to shape his or her stance on current topics. When a new issue comes up, the health legislative assistant pulls together information to make sure the legislator is informed. He or she meets with stakeholders, such as health advocacy organizations, gives formal presentations, and may draft new bills related to health issues. The job can include preparing speeches for the legislator and helping him or her prepare for media interviews. Legislative assistants also respond to questions from individual constituents and talk with members of the press. Often, a legislative assistant who handles health issues also covers other topic areas, dividing his or her time among multiple subjects. This job can be very fast-paced and stressful, and can require long hours.

Education and Certification

The requirements for this job differ according to the legislator's expectations and needs. There are jobs for people just starting out after college who have had policy-related internships or some experience on Capitol Hill. And there are jobs that require significant expertise, with previous

Congressional experience or a strong policy background. Some come to this job from a policy analyst role; some come from industry; some come from a clinical background with training in public health or health policy. Many have an MPH, an MPP, or a master's in health management and policy.

Core Competencies and Skills

- Ability to work under pressure and willingness to work long hours
- Ability to multitask
- Good attention to detail
- Ability to analyze information, determine what is most relevant, and present the information in a concise and logical way
- Ability to work under pressure and to meet tight deadlines
- Good political judgment and an understanding of how the legislative process works
- Understanding of health policy issues, including Medicare, Medicaid, and insurance reform

Compensation

A legislative assistant in the House or Senate often starts out in the low $30,000s to mid $40,000s, with compensation increasing with expertise and experience. In 2006, average salaries were about $67,000 in the Senate and $43,000 in the House. The top possible salary for a legislative assistant in the Senate is about $160,000, but it is rare that one would earn that much.

Workplaces

There are legislative assistants at both state and federal levels. Legislators at the state level usually have fewer staff members than senators and representatives in Washington, DC, and are less likely to have designated assistants focusing on health.

Employment Outlook

There is a lot of turnover in these jobs, both because people often use them as steppingstones to other opportunities, and because of changes following elections. It means that jobs are available fairly regularly. However, there is also a lot of competition for each position. Doing an internship at a legislative office and taking advantage of networking opportunities can be good way to get in the door.

For Further Information

- Congressional Legislative Staff Association (CLSA) *www.uscongressionalstaff.org*
- National Conference of State Legislatures (NCSL) *www.ncsl.org*

HEALTH ECONOMIST

Job Description

A health economist uses specialized knowledge of economics and finance to promote sound health policy. A health economist might focus specifically on the economic effects of policies such as a national health care plan. He or she might help an organization or agency decide which public health programs are most financially sound or cost effective. Some economists help evaluate health technology. Some assess the cost effectiveness of different treatment options. Economists also help evaluate existing programs to see if money is being wasted. Overall, the role often includes tracking down data on economic indicators, analyzing trends over time, and developing models to predict the future balance between costs and health benefits. This is usually a desk job with a lot of computer time, but it can also involve creative problem solving and the opportunity to have a direct impact on policy.

Education and Certification

A bachelor's degree in economics is the absolute minimum educational requirement. Opportunities beyond entry-level jobs often require a master's degree, and a PhD is the standard for a health economist who leads a team or a project.

Core Competencies and Skills

- Interest in health policy and a thorough understanding of economics as applied to health care

- Ability to sort through information and decide what elements are most relevant
- Strong written and verbal communication skills, including the ability to explain the work to non-economists
- Persistence and patience for projects that take significant time to complete
- Knowledge of economic issues in relevant fields such as health insurance, medical technology, pharmaceuticals, or hospital finance
- Strong statistical knowledge and analytical skills and a high level of comfort with math and numbers

Compensation

The median salary for all economists was about $84,000 per year in 2008. Most earned between $44,000 and $149,000.

Workplaces

Health economists serve the cause of public health in city, county, and state governments, at federal agencies (including CDC, NIH, CMS, and the Government Accountability Office), and at nonprofits, think tanks, and consulting firms. There are also health economists doing cost-effectiveness research at pharmaceutical companies and insurance companies.

Employment Outlook

Compared to the national average for all occupations, employment of economists is expected to grow relatively slowly through 2010. However, people who are well qualified as health economists tend to be in demand for this specialized job. With cost-effectiveness becoming an increasingly important concern, opportunities may actually expand over the next several years.

For Further Information

See the Policy Analyst description. Also:

- American Society of Health Economists (ASHEcon) *healtheconomics.us*

PUBLIC HEALTH LAWYER

Job Description

A public health lawyer uses legal expertise to assist with efforts to safeguard and promote the public's health. At a health department or federal agency such as the CDC, a public health lawyer gives advice to policymakers and reviews plans and policies to identify potential pitfalls. Can the government require every doctor to get a flu shot? If city officials want restaurants to post calorie information, how should the policy be worded, and what legal challenges might come up? A significant part of the work at state and local agencies has to do with regulatory matters, for example, looking at the legal aspects of creating ordinances to limit indoor air pollution. Another typical role is helping defend patient confidentiality. Public health lawyers handle lawsuits against public health agencies, as well, and help fight challenges to laws that protect people's health and safety. Some public health lawyers help nonprofits and community organizations take full advantage of existing laws and regulations. For example, they can figure out how to use economic development resources to get public land set aside for a community garden.

Education and Certification

A public health lawyer needs a law degree, a license to practice, and knowledge of public health law, which can be obtained through education or practice. Many public health lawyers have an MPH in addition to the JD.

Core Competencies and Skills

- Commitment to serving the public and a passion for public health
- Persuasiveness
- Ability to explain legal principles to nonlawyers
- Understanding of the legal framework for public health, including government agencies' roles and the scope of states' powers
- Awareness of issues in public health ethics
- Knowledge regarding the areas of public health that the work will address

Compensation

In the profession as a whole, most lawyers earn between $54,000 and $163,000. The median salary is about $111,000. Public health lawyers tend to earn less than lawyers with similar levels of experience in private practice or industry.

Workplaces

Public health lawyers work for the government and for nonprofit and political organizations. At the state and local levels, they are usually at the health department or the attorney general's office; there are also public health lawyers at federal agencies. Some lawyers with public health knowledge work in industry, advising corporate leaders about what government agencies might do and how best to work with them. Some public health lawyers work in academia; public health law research is an emerging field.

Employment Outlook

There is significant competition for job openings for lawyers, including those that are directed toward public service. The Bureau of Labor Services predicts that, overall, there will continue to be more lawyers than available jobs. However, there may be increasing opportunities in public health law in the future, as politics and health become more intertwined.

For Further Information

- Public Health Law Association (PHLA)
  www.phla.info
- Centers for Disease Control and Prevention—Public Health Law Program (PHLP)
  www2.cdc.gov/phlp
- The American Society of Law, Medicine, and Ethics (ASLME)
  www.aslme.org
- The Centers for Law and the Public's Health
  www.publichealthlaw.net

ADMINISTRATIVE LAW JUDGE

Job Description

Administrative law judges conduct hearings and make rulings in cases having to do with so-called administrative issues, such as the enforcement of health and safety regulations. When a doctor is accused of professional misconduct, the administrative law judge hears the case and makes recommendations for disciplinary action. An administrative law judge might hear an appeal by a woman who has been denied WIC coverage, or make a judgment about a violation of the sanitary code. A case of a store selling cigarettes to children would go to the administrative law judge, as well. These judges' tasks include holding conferences before official hearings, issuing subpoenas, conducting hearings, listening to oral testimony or reading written documents, and issuing written findings and decisions. State administrative law judges may have significant amounts of travel, as they go to hear cases in different regions. They usually have 8-hour workdays and weekends off.

Education and Certification

Becoming an administrative law judge at the federal level requires a law degree and a specific examination set by the U.S. Office of Personnel Management. At the state level, a law degree may or may not be required. Some departments require a certain level of experience practicing law.

Core Competencies and Skills

- Fairness
- Logical thinking
- Patience and good listening skills
- Excellent problem-solving ability
- Good time management skills
- Strong understanding of public health law and health department regulations
- Knowledge of court procedures and related rules and regulations
- Ability to understand multiple points of view

Compensation

The median salary for administrative law judges and hearing officers was about $77,000 in 2008. Most earned between $37,000 and $140,000.

Workplaces

Administrative law judges who hear health-related cases are employed at the state and federal levels and by some cities and counties. An administrative law judge may work directly for a health department or for a separate agency that focuses on administrative law hearings. Administrative law judges at state environmental agencies sometimes hear health-related cases, too. In federal government, administrative law judges work for many agencies including HHS.

Employment Outlook

Administrative law judge is a civil service job, which provides some job security. National statistics for employment outlook cover all types of judges, not just administrative law judges; in general, employee turnover tends to be low and there is competition for available jobs. However, pay is higher in the private sector, and this may lessen competition.

For Further Information

- The National Association of Administrative Law Judiciary (NAALJ) *www.naalj.org*
- National Association of Hearing Officials (NAHO) *www.naho.org*
- National Conference of the Administrative Law Judiciary *new.abanet.org/divisions/judicial/ncalj/Pages/default.aspx*

CONSUMER ADVOCATE

Job Description

"Consumer advocate," like "activist," is a title that can represent many different jobs. But essentially, a consumer advocate is someone who helps people obtain safe products and fair services. Consumer advocates don't necessarily focus on health, but those who do help protect the public from products that could cause injury and from inadequate medical care. There are consumer advocates working to improve the laws and regulations that govern the safety of consumer products, pharmaceuticals, or medical devices. Some focus on health insurance restrictions or on the quality of care at hospitals and doctors' offices. They track down data on product- or service-related injuries, read current laws and policies, and write reports and recommendations based on this information. They speak with industry executives, give testimony at legislative hearings, talk to reporters, and meet with people from the community and from other advocacy organizations. Some consumer advocates make regular appearances on television and radio. Consumer advocates may also lead grassroots efforts to encourage consumers to take a stand themselves, or they may use legal skills to go after manufacturers who make harmful products.

Education and Certification

Educational needs differ according to the job. A consumer advocate may be a lawyer, a policy or public health expert, a community organizer, or simply an ordinary citizen with the zeal, persistence, and networking skills to get things done.

Core Competencies and Skills

- Passion for public safety and consumers' rights
- Excellent communication skills, including public speaking skills
- Persuasiveness
- Ability to select information that will gain the attention of reporters, policymakers, and the public
- Understanding of laws and policies related to consumer safety
- Understanding of the political process

Compensation

Salaries depend greatly on the type of organization and type of work. A small grassroots organization might pay as little as $25,000 to $30,000, while someone with significant experience at a large organization could earn $100,000 or more.

Workplaces

Many consumer advocates work for nonprofit advocacy organizations. Some states have a "consumer advocate" office that deals with insurance issues, including health insurance; these offices handle complaints against insurance companies and may also offer consumer education. There are jobs for people interested in consumer protection at federal agencies including the Federal Trade Commission (FTC) and the Consumer Product Safety Commission (CPSC); there are opportunities for inspectors, program analysts, attorneys, and others.

Employment Outlook

Jobs at advocacy organizations will likely expand a bit faster than the national average from 2008 through 2018. Because these jobs tend to have lower wages than jobs in the for-profit sector, there is significant turnover. There have been budget cuts at CPSC in recent years, although there are usually several job openings listed at USAjobs.gov; the number of future opportunities will depend on funding of the agency.

For Further Information

- Center for Science in the Public Interest (CSPI)
  www.cspinet.org
- Consumers Union (CU)
  www.consumersunion.org
- Public Citizen
  www.citizen.org
- Consumer Federation of America (CFA)
  www.consumerfed.org
- National Consumers League (NCL)
  www.nclnet.org

PUBLIC HEALTH LOBBYIST

Job Description

A lobbyist's job is to influence legislators to make decisions that support his client's interests. Traditionally, lobbying is thought of as interacting directly with legislators and their staff members, to persuade them to pass a favorable law, or prevent passage of a damaging one. Lobbyists contribute to political debate by sharing information and perspectives from the groups they represent. There is also grassroots lobbying, which involves enlisting the help of the public, such as organizing rallies or demonstrations, or asking people to call their Congressman.

A lobbyist for an organization concerned with public health will have face-to-face meetings with legislators, legislative assistants, and influential government officials. The lobbyist observes relevant legislative hearings and sometimes offers official testimony. He or she might arrange for organization members to visit Washington, DC, or a state capitol and meet with legislators. The job requires keeping up with the news and new developments, as well as finding out about legislators' political interests, tracking how they plan to vote, and looking for approaches they will find persuasive. The lobbyist may also be tasked with persuading state and federal agencies to create regulations that support his or her organization's cause. This job may require long hours and travel. A lobbyist's job description can overlap with that of an organization's advocacy director.

Education and Certification

A lobbyist will usually have at least a bachelor's degree and some experience in the political world. Many have master's degrees or law degrees.

Core Competencies and Skills

- Excellent interpersonal and networking skills
- Persuasiveness and strong negotiation skills
- Excellent organizational skills
- Ability to work independently, to meet deadlines, and to handle stress
- Good understanding of politics
- Familiarity with medical and public health issues
- Knowledge of how laws are passed and regulations are created
- Understanding of public relations and media

Compensation

Lobbyists who work for industry can earn very comfortable salaries. According to nationwide survey data, the average salary for a lobbyist is about $97,000, and those with extensive experience or strong credentials can earn a great deal more. Health advocacy organizations tend to have smaller budgets than industry, however, and nonprofits can spend only a limited amount on lobbying. Some lobbyists working on social issues earn salaries more in the range of $50,000.

Workplaces

Most lobbyists work in large cities, particularly Washington, DC. They may be employed directly by organizations and associations concerned with health issues, or they may work for lobbying firms or other private companies that contract with such organizations. A public health lobbyist may work for multiple organizations, each with a limited budget, or do this work as part of another job.

Employment Outlook

The Bureau of Labor Statistics does not offer outlook data for lobbying jobs. The American League of Lobbyists suggests that people interested in entering this career look for experience, even an internship, in a congressional office. Another option is to begin doing public relations and advocacy work for an organization and then look for opportunities to focus on lobbying. Lobbying skills can also translate to other policy-related careers.

For Further Information

■ American League of Lobbyists (ALL)
  www.alldc.org
■ Also see the Web sites in the description for advocacy director.

REFERENCES

Gostin, L. O. (2001). *Public health law: Power, duty, and restraint.* Los Angeles: University of California Press.

Wing, K. R., & Gilbert, B. (2007). *The law and the public's health* (7th ed.). Chicago: Health Administration Press.

18 Evaluation, Safety, and Quality

The careers in this chapter focus on making sure that both public health and individual health care services are accomplishing what we want and expect them to do.

Historically, funding for the evaluation of many public health programs was limited or nonexistent. Now, funders often expect programs to include evaluation, and government agencies require that programs be based on scientific evidence whenever possible. Slowly, public health is building up a base of evidence that can be used to design future programs for maximum impact.

Health care quality and patient safety are also gaining in importance, as we recognize that there are significant problems in these areas. Modern patient safety practices encourage health care providers to report errors, analyze the causes, and look for ways to improve systems so that patient safety errors are unlikely to recur.

Health care quality includes the effectiveness of the care that doctors, nurses, dentists, and other health professionals provide. The goal of health care quality efforts is to improve the health of our population by identifying, solving, and preventing problems in the delivery of care.

Those interested in the connection between medical care and public health can get involved with the APHA section on Medical Care, at www.apha.org.

Many public health jobs include elements of evaluation or quality improvement. Infection control specialists are concerned with one element of patient safety. Other related jobs include medical epidemiologist, hospital administrator, and pharmacist.

PROGRAM EVALUATOR

Job Description

A program evaluator is responsible for determining if a public health program is accomplishing what it was designed to do. This includes how the program is being run, whether it is properly designed, how services are being delivered, and—most important—whether the program is making a difference. Sometimes program evaluators are involved in planning public health projects, as well. If you want to know whether a bike safety campaign got more people to wear helmets, you need to know what percentage of people were using helmets in the first place. Then, you need to be able to measure how many people changed their behavior and whether they did so because of the campaign or for some other reason. Program evaluators can give advice about how to collect this information in the most accurate, efficient way.

Specific tasks might include researching medical information, determining exactly what data will be most informative, and creating surveys. Once a program is underway, an evaluator might monitor staff performance, look at preliminary results, and keep an eye on how well the effort is working. If the program has a set end date, the evaluator collects and analyzes information about the final result. Throughout the process, the evaluator reports back to the people who run the program, to the funders, or to others. This job can include a lot of computer time, doing data analysis and writing reports, but it can also involve visits to program sites and interacting with staff and participants.

Education and Certification

This job requires training in program evaluation or related knowledge and experience. MPH, MPA, or MPP coursework can provide the necessary skills. Some senior-level and leadership positions require a PhD. Research or program planning experience can sometimes take the place of specific evaluation training, but an understanding of statistics and data analysis, including how to use statistics programs on a computer, is essential. Some schools offer a non-degree certificate in program evaluation. It is also possible to earn a master's degree in program evaluation, although this is usually associated with another course of study such as psychology or education.

Core Competencies and Skills

- Good organizational skills
- Analytical thinking
- Ability to work within time constraints
- Familiarity with quality improvement techniques
- Ability to summarize findings for different types of audiences
- Knowledge of statistical techniques used in program evaluation
- Familiarity with public health programs in general and with the type of program being evaluated
- Ability to use computer programs to run statistical analyses and to create charts and graphs

Compensation

According to a 2006 salary survey, compensation can range from a nominal amount to well over $100,000. The majority of evaluators earned between $30,000 and $100,000, and the most common salaries were in the $40,000 to $70,000 range.

Workplaces

Public health program evaluators do their work at government agencies, nonprofits, universities, and consulting firms.

Employment Outlook

The public health world has been paying increasing attention to program evaluation, and funders often require evaluation plans in grant proposals. *U.S. News and World Report* included this job in a 2009 list of little-known careers with good prospects for employment.

For Further Information

- American Evaluation Association (AEA)
  www.eval.org

PUBLIC HEALTH PROFILE: Program Evaluator
Allison Meserve, MPH
Research Associate
Public Health Solutions, New York, NY

Describe the sort of work you do.

I work for a nonprofit organization. We have over 600 employees, whose responsibilities include running WIC centers, early intervention programs and reproductive health clinics; offering consulting services and technical assistance for nonprofits; and distributing grant money for programs that provide care for people with HIV.

I work in the research and evaluation unit. We evaluate programs to determine if they are meeting goals during the process and then to determine the impact of the project. My main focus is reproductive health issues, like contraceptive choice.

What is a typical day like at your job?

Most of my time is spent with program data or research data, getting it ready for analysis, analyzing it, and writing reports about it. A smaller part of what I do is pre- and post-program development—figuring out what indicators we should track, then what worked well and what didn't, and what recommendations we should make for the future. Occasionally, I go to our clinics to supervise the research being done. My major project right now is an evaluation of a computer module that suggests birth control methods to fit individual women's needs. Later today, I'll be looking at some data from an online survey that we did with men who have sex with men. I'll also be doing a literature review for a grant proposal we are going to write for another research project.

What education or training do you have? Is it typical for your job?

I have an MPH degree. My undergraduate major was women's studies. Some people doing monitoring and evaluation have another type of master's degree, but for public health work it is better to have an

Continued

MPH because you'll understand the issues and the literature. You also need to have experience with data analysis and statistics programs, which you can get as part of your MPH training. For higher-level jobs in project evaluation, you need a doctoral degree.

What path did you take to get to the job you are in today?

When I was in college, I thought I was going to go to medical school but after taking a few classes on women's issues in developing countries, I decided I wanted to go into international development. I spent 4 years in Mali.

My personal life led me back to the United States. I decided to get my MPH, and I learned about my current job when I was working for a professor in my MPH program. She heard about this position, and she emailed my current boss and said, "I know a great candidate!" This job involves a really interesting patient population, mostly immigrants, so it is a way for me to still be involved with people from different backgrounds.

Where might you go from here, if you wanted to advance your career?

When I think about next steps, I'm thinking several years from now. I could probably stay in program evaluation, possibly moving to an organization that wants an in-house evaluator, which would give me more responsibility. I've also considered running a nonprofit organization. I have the program and finance background from my previous work, and the monitoring and evaluation experience is a nice addition.

What is the worst or most challenging part of your job?

The most frustrating part is trying to translate for people who don't have experience with evaluation. I have to explain why certain things are important. Often people want to use anecdotal evidence, and it can be hard to explain why that is not enough.

What is the best part?

On the contraceptive choice project I've been working on, it is nice to see that a module we designed is actually making a difference in

Continued

women's contraceptive choices and their reproductive lives. One of the things we see is that the methods they're interested in are not the most effective. We hope that this module will help them choose more effective ones.

What advice do you have for someone who is interested in your career?

Take classes in quantitative and qualitative analysis, but also make sure you are getting actual work experience that uses those skills. A lot of people graduating with an MPH are going to have taken the same classes, so you'll have an advantage if you can show that you have been responsible for data analysis. Also, try to learn about how programs really function. The fact that I've worked in public health programs makes it easier for me to interact with program staff. I know how hard it can be for them to get things done with time and budget constraints.

QUALITY IMPROVEMENT SPECIALIST

Job Description

A quality improvement specialist works either as a consultant or within an organization to make the organization function better. That can include making the organization more efficient, improving the way services are delivered, or improving the services themselves. The goal could be providing safer care throughout a hospital, increasing the number of adults who receive the flu vaccine, or streamlining health inspections so that more restaurants can be checked each month. Quality improvement experts begin by figuring out where improvements are needed. Next, they study organizational culture and the systems that are currently in place. They do what they can to gain the cooperation of employees and to work with them to decide what steps to take. Then, they help implement changes, monitor results, and continue to work with staff members to adjust plans as needed. If an organization has to follow certain government regulations or medical guidelines, quality improvement also means making sure the rules are being followed.

Education and Certification

These jobs usually require a bachelor's or master's degree, with relevant training or experience. The coursework for an MPH or MPA typically includes training in quality improvement, and an MPH is the preferred training for some jobs. There are also quality improvement jobs that require a doctoral degree, such as a PhD or MD, because specialized knowledge is needed to understand the training offered, services provided, or outcomes. Some jobs require a nursing degree or other clinical training. There are opportunities for general quality improvement certification through organizations such as the American Society for Quality; the National Association for Healthcare Quality has a certification for professionals in clinical care quality management.

Core Competencies and Skills

- Good presentation skills
- Good understanding of human nature
- Good understanding of how workplace and health care systems work and where they are likely to break down
- Knowledge of quality improvement theory and techniques
- Understanding of program evaluation principles
- At least basic skills in statistics
- Ability to use computer programs to create charts and graphs

Compensation

It is difficult to give a typical salary for a quality improvement specialist, because salaries depend on the size and type of the organization and the level of expertise needed. According to data compiled by the Web site salary.com, a typical health care quality improvement director might expect to earn $76,000 to $131,000, while a head nurse in charge of quality improvement might earn $53,000 to $77,000. A recent opening for a quality improvement specialist with a bachelor's degree and some experience offered a range of $39,000 to $59,000.

Workplaces

Quality improvement specialists work for all sorts of health-related organizations and government agencies. There are jobs at health departments, at consulting firms, and at Quality Improvement Organizations (QIOs). (QIOs are organizations, usually nonprofits, that contract with the CMS to work on improving the quality of Medicare.) Many hospitals and health care systems hire specialists who use public health techniques to improve direct care.

Employment Outlook

There are often job openings in direct-care settings. In more traditional public health settings, quality improvement can be a separate full-time job, but it is frequently part of a broader job description. There are indications of increasing interest that could lead to new opportunities, however, if funding is available. For example, the National Association of City and County Health Officials (NACCHO) is planning a voluntary accreditation system for health departments, to be launched in 2011, that will include a quality improvement element.

For Further Information

- American Health Quality Association (AHQA)
  www.ahqa.org
- American Society for Quality (ASQ)
  www.asq.org
- Agency for Healthcare Research and Quality (AHRQ)
  www.ahrq.gov

OUTCOMES RESEARCHER

Job Description

An outcomes researcher studies the results of health care practices and interventions. This means measuring not just, say, how many people got the right medicines after a heart attack, but how long those people lived afterwards and whether they had good quality of life. It means looking at treatment for pneumonia in the hospital compared to treatment at home, to see if the less expensive home option can save Medicare money without compromising patients' health or safety. Outcomes research can also identify practices that aren't helpful—and sometimes, it even catches treatments that are causing harm. Collecting outcomes information can be challenging. How do you follow up on patients after they have left the hospital? Outcomes researchers work with clinicians to decide what information is important and how to gather it. They organize the data, decide the best way to analyze it, and carry out the analysis. Then, they present the results to stakeholders. Outcomes researchers may also be involved in writing grant proposals, writing scientific papers, and presenting at conferences. There is a lot of numbers-crunching and computer time in this job, plus communications and meetings with stakeholders.

Education and Certification

Because of the level of knowledge required, including experience with original research, many of these jobs require a doctoral-level degree or at least a master's in public health, epidemiology, or a related field. Most important is having training or experience in this type of research, and experience with managed care institutions or the pharmaceutical industry is often helpful.

Core Competencies and Skills

- Strong study design and statistical analysis skills
- Good organizational skills
- Proficiency with computer programs for statistical analysis
- Understanding of how patient data are collected and reported
- Strong creative problem-solving skills
- Ability to work with both clinical personnel and administrators
- Ability to translate research results into a language and format that nonexperts can understand

Compensation

People who do outcomes research are often classed as biostatisticians, epidemiologists, health scientists, or medical officers. There are no national salary statistics for this job title, but here are some examples. A physician serving as a researcher at a federal agency, with some leadership responsibility, might earn between $100,000 and $130,000. An opening for an experienced health services researcher at NCI, with PhD-level training and supervisory responsibilities, offers a range of $87,000 to $134,000.

Workplaces

Outcomes researchers work at government agencies, at hospitals and health systems including the Veterans Administration, in academia, and for private consulting or research firms. Pharmaceutical manufacturers are also a major employer of outcomes researchers; there are public health aspects to these jobs, but the ultimate intention tends more toward improving marketing and sales.

Employment Outlook

Again, national statistics are lacking, but there is significant interest in outcomes and in the related field of cost-effectiveness research within the agencies of HHS.

For Further Information

- Agency for Healthcare and Quality (AHRQ)
  www.ahrq.gov
- Society for Medical Decision Making (SMDM)
  www.smdm.org
- International Society for Pharmacoeconomics and Outcomes Research (ISPOR)
  www.ispor.org

INFORMATICS SPECIALIST

Job Description

Informatics is about the collection, organization, storage, classification, and retrieval of information. "Public health informatics," specifically, uses computer science and technology to facilitate public health research, practice, and education. Informatics specialists might look at how to integrate disease surveillance data from different systems, how to help public health officials share information in an emergency, or how to have public health alerts appear automatically in electronic medical records systems. There is also a significant role for informatics in health services research, making use of patient data to reveal spending patterns, flag infection risks, or track patient safety. Informatics specialists handle complex organizational and computing challenges on a regular basis. For example, a single surveillance system can bring together hundreds of thousands of data points from laboratories, hospitals, other health care facilities, and individual doctors. This job typically involves a lot of computer time and has standard business hours, although tricky problems or tight deadlines can sometimes require staying late.

Education and Certification

Training requirements vary, particularly because this is a relatively new field. There are jobs for people with bachelor's degrees, but these are usually at an assistant level. More interesting and challenging jobs require at least a master's degree, such as an MPH with an informatics focus. Some jobs involving electronic medical records require a nursing or medical degree. Advancement can be through education, experience, or both. In addition to degree programs, as of 2010 there are training opportunities in public health informatics at the CDC and in medical informatics through the NIH.

Core Competencies and Skills

- Excellent computer skills, including programming knowledge and knowledge of available hardware and software
- Strong organizational skills, not just for job tasks but also for information
- Interest in solving complicated problems
- Understanding of how people use databases and information systems, and of how to create systems that are intuitive to use
- Ability to communicate with people who are experts in other fields, and who may not be computer-savvy
- Understanding of relevant public health or medical issues

Compensation

The U.S. Bureau of Labor Statistics doesn't track informatics as a separate job title. Bachelor's degree graduates can expect starting salaries of about $40,000 to $50,000. An experienced leader of an informatics team at a large agency or consulting firm, with a master's degree or a PhD, could earn $150,000 to $200,000. A 2008 survey by the Healthcare Information and Management Systems Society, including people with many different job titles and level of experience, found a median salary of $96,000.

Workplaces

The CDC has a National Center for Public Health Informatics, which also supports several Centers of Excellence in Public Health Informatics at universities throughout the United States. There are informatics specialists working in other areas of the CDC and other agencies within HHS, at health departments, at other universities, at nonprofits concerned with public health or global health, and at private consulting firms. Hospitals, medical centers, and consulting firms employ informatics specialists to work on electronic medical records systems, and HHS has Regional Extension Centers to provide technical assistance to health care providers establishing electronic medical records.

Employment Outlook

This is a fast-growing field. There should be very good opportunities in informatics as more and more health care systems move to electronic medical records, and as the CDC and other health agencies continue to build and improve public health information systems.

For Further Information

- American Medical Informatics Association (AMIA)
  www.amia.org
- Healthcare Information and Management Systems Society (HIMSS)
  www.himss.org
- American Public Health Association—Health Informatics Information Technology section
  www.apha.org/membergroups/sections/aphasections/hiit
- CDC Public Health Informatics Network (PHIN)
  www.cdc.gov/phin

PATIENT SAFETY SPECIALIST

Job Description

Patient safety specialists track reports about safety hazards at hospitals, medical centers, doctors' offices, or pharmacies. Instead of focusing on individual errors, they look for places within the system where mistakes or problems are likely to occur. This could include opportunities for nurses to give the wrong medication by accident, for patients to slip and fall, or for doctors to overlook abnormal lab results. They investigate incidents, and they work with clinical teams to figure out whether systematic changes—such as flagging lab results in a more obvious way, or adding extra safeguards on medication dispensing—could prevent future problems. They recommend specific changes when necessary. Then, they follow up to see if plans have been implemented and safety has improved. Patient safety specialists also assess systems to look for places where problems could occur, even if nothing has gone wrong yet.

Some health departments have their own patient safety specialists who work with local health care providers to track incidents and encourage good safety practices. The job combines deskwork with presentations and visits to various clinical departments to observe current practices.

Education and Certification

Patient safety specialists in hospitals are usually, but not always, registered nurses. A master's degree (such as an MSN or MPH), with training in patient safety and quality management, is often preferred. The Certified Professional in Health Quality credential can be helpful. Health departments sometimes look for people with PhDs or MPH degrees to oversee local patient safety efforts. However, there is no single, specific educational pathway.

Core Competencies and Skills

- Computer skills, including databases and presentation software
- Confidence in public speaking and presenting information
- Knowledge of quality improvement techniques
- Understanding of at least basic epidemiology and statistics
- Knowledge of safety regulations
- Knowledge of national patient safety organizations and initiatives
- Familiarity with health information, including clinical knowledge and awareness of how the health care system works

Compensation

Patient safety specialists earn about $41,000 to $73,000 per year, according to national data from salary.com.

Workplaces

Patient safety specialists are usually found in hospitals and large health care systems. There are also people working on patient safety at health departments and at nonprofit organizations.

Employment Outlook

There should be good opportunities for nurses in this field. People without clinical degrees will have a harder time finding hands-on patient safety work, but there are opportunities for people with public health training to get involved in patient safety in other ways, such as an analyst role.

For Further Information

- Agency for Healthcare Research and Quality (AHRQ)
  www.ahrq.gov
- National Patient Safety Foundation (NPSF)
  www.npsf.org
- National Academy for State Health Policy (NASHP)
  www.nashp.org
- Institute for Healthcare Improvement (IHI)
  www.ihi.org

PUBLIC HEALTH PROFILE: Patient Safety Specialist
Iona Thraen, ACSW, PhD Candidate
Director, Patient Safety Initiative
Utah Department of Health, Salt Lake City, UT

Describe the sort of work you do.

My job is to develop Utah's patient safety program and to liaise with health care industry representatives, including pharmacists, hospital administrators, risk managers, quality managers, and infection control practitioners. I collect information, analyze data, and work with industry representatives to devise interventions, tools and other resources that will improve the safety of care. We have developed a web-based error reporting system and I'm working on ways to integrate the patient safety initiative with other parts of the health department.

Continued

What is a typical day like at your job?

Yesterday started with a rule revision committee meeting. We have a set of rules for reporting intravenous line infections in ICUs, and now we're looking at creating a set of rules for reporting another type of hospital-associated infection. We were talking about creating an umbrella approach, with a single rule for reporting multiple types of infections instead of separate rules for each one. Later, I met with executives from the health department to report on patient safety activities. On other days I might meet with our infectious disease epidemiologists to talk about infections that occur in hospitals, or work with the neonatal screening program on assuring blood specimens from hospitals are submitted in a timely fashion. I also spend time writing reports on patient safety issues and preparing presentations.

Recently, I presented data to our Patient Safety Users group, which includes hospital representatives, the Utah Hospital Association, the Department of Health, and our region's QIO. At those group meetings we also discuss upcoming projects, in terms of where to focus our efforts and resources.

What education or training do you have? Is it typical for your job?

A lot of people doing patient safety work are nurses. I have a bachelor's in psychology, a master's in social work, and some graduate work in health care economics. I'm now working on a PhD in medical informatics and social work. To me, this job is less about specific clinical expertise than about consensus building and process: getting people to agree to report errors, finding the best way for them to do that, and using the data from the reports to create change and improve the safety of care.

What path did you take to get to the job you are in today?

Since moving to Utah, I spent a year with a QIO as a project manager, and then I was the administrator for a small nonprofit that had gotten a Robert Wood Johnson Foundation grant to work with rural hospitals on quality improvement. I was recruited to the health department as a division director, and later patient safety was added to my responsibilities. When there was a change in political leadership I used the

Continued

opportunity to propose a half-time position dedicated exclusively to patient safety. At first they said no, and I was prepared to leave and take another job—but then they changed their minds. The job has since expanded to 35 hours per week.

Where might you go from here, if you wanted to advance your career?

For me, completing a PhD in medical informatics is a means to an end. The way in which we collect data today is a manual, voluntary reporting system, and only a small fraction of medical errors are reported each year. Its not that they're being hidden, necessarily, but they often don't show up on the radar screen. The future for health care quality and patient safety is in electronic medical records and automated reporting. I would like to be the liaison between the information technology staff and the clinical staff, making sure that we capture and use data in such a way that we can prevent errors and create better safeguards.

What is the worst or most challenging part of your job?

Before we had the web-based reporting system, I had to enter data by hand. Developing administrative regulations and rules can also be tedious, because it takes a lot of going back and forth with attorneys and a lot of legalese.

What is the best part?

The best part is that patient safety is a fairly new domain, and so I'm constantly learning. We are all still learning about how to improve patient safety and figuring out how to create new systems.

What advice do you have for someone who is interested in your career?

Patient safety is a rapidly changing field. What is going on today may not be happening a few years from now. There was no patient safety position at the health department 10 years ago—I created this job! So keep in mind that the field of public health evolves and changes, and you have to keep current and change with it. People worry about age discrimination—but I'll be 60 years old when I graduate with my PhD, and I'll be one of the most currently trained people in the marketplace.

HEALTH FACILITY SURVEYOR

Job Description

A health facility surveyor visits nursing homes, other long-term or residential care facilities, dialysis centers, and other health care settings to verify that they are following state and federal regulations, and sometimes to investigate complaints. The surveyor travels to the facility, where he or she observes the staff and speaks with patients. The surveyor reviews medical records, examines administrative policies and procedures, and looks at other documents and records as needed to make sure that the facility is complying with regulations and providing appropriate care. Surveyors who are clinically trained also examine patients for signs of maltreatment or improper care. In some positions, the surveyor's role extends to inspecting the fire safety systems, as well. The surveyor shares his or her findings, including any violations, with the facility management, and writes an official report. When legal cases arise, the surveyor's report may be subpoenaed, and he or she will occasionally need to testify at a hearing. Some health facility surveyors also help with provider training, assist facilities in doing what is needed to meet requirements, and take part in planning when changes to state regulations are needed. The job can involve overnight travel to facilities throughout a region or state.

Education and Certification

Health facility surveyors are often nurses, who must be licensed to practice. Many employers prefer applicants with experience providing patient care in a facility like the ones being inspected. Depending on the specific job, a surveyor may, instead, have a bachelor's or higher degree in a relevant field such as public health or hospital administration, plus experience with health care administration or inspection. Some surveyor jobs require training and certification in more specific fields such as nutrition or environmental health. Surveyors who inspect long-term care facilities that receive money from Medicare and Medicaid must also pass the federal Surveyor Minimum Qualifications Test either before or within a set time after beginning work.

Core Competencies and Skills

- Understanding of proper medical record-keeping and appropriate care

- Willingness to travel
- Good "people skills," including the ability to give criticism honestly but tactfully
- Excellent observational skills
- Physical ability to be on your feet and moving all day
- Ability to work both independently and as part of a team
- Writing skills that are adequate to convey findings, plus the ability to translate between medical jargon and plain English
- Ability to use state computer programs for making reports or entering data

Compensation

Health care surveyors earn about $25,000 to $70,000 per year, depending on experience and location. The higher-paid jobs, for surveyors with more experience, often involve supervisory and management tasks.

Workplaces

Surveyors work for state health departments or regulatory agencies. There are also regional CMS offices that oversee and provide guidance to state certification agencies. Some private companies employ surveyors to do "practice" inspections and help health care facilities ensure they are meeting regulations.

Employment Outlook

Employment of surveyors will likely be stable, as there is an ongoing need for this type of work.

For Further Information

- Centers for Medicare & Medicaid Services (CMS)
  www.cms.gov

REFERENCE

Kohn, L. T., Corrigan, J. M., & Donaldson, M. S. (2000). *To err is human: Building a safer health system.* Washington, DC: National Academy Press.

Nonprofit Organizations

Nonprofit organizations serve an important purpose in public health. There are nonprofits providing policy analysis and synthesizing information about vital public health issues. Nonprofits advocate for policy change related to cancer prevention, the prevention of violence, workplace safety, and more. There are foundations that provide large amounts of funding for research projects and public programs, shaping the picture of public health both locally and nationwide.

The jobs in this section are not unique to public health; they're found in nonprofits of all types. They're included here both as a reminder of the role of nonprofits in promoting health and preventing disease, and as an introduction to some of the careers in these helpful organizations.

GRANT WRITER

Job Description

A lot of public health work is funded by grants from nonprofit organizations or from state or federal government agencies. Grant writers create the applications, often called "grant proposals," that tell funders about a project and invite them to support it. A grant writer begins the work on each proposal by learning about the organization or program that is seeking funds. The writer seeks out information about the potential funder and looks for ways that the organization's and the funder's goals might coincide, so that he or she can present the program in the best possible light. The writer checks the funder's requirements for the proposal and follows the specified structure. Most grant proposals include details about the project, its goals, the evidence behind it, the people involved, the timeline, and the budget. There will usually be some back-and-forth between the writer and the program planners or other leaders at the organization or agency seeking funds, to ensure that the proposal matches what is really planned. In some cases, the grant writer also helps locate potential funding sources and stays in touch with them after the grant proposal has been submitted, in case additional information is needed.

Education and Certification

Excellent writing skills and a sense of what will appeal to funders are the most important qualifications. Most grant writers have at least a bachelor's degree and many have advanced degrees. Advanced knowledge of science, medicine, or public health can be helpful if the grant has to do with a complex health issue. For those who want specific training, several schools offer certificate programs in grant writing. There are also optional professional certifications from the American Association of Grant Professionals and the American Grant Writers' Association.

Core Competencies and Skills

- Ability to learn new information quickly
- Ability to meet deadlines
- Strong writing skills, with a high level of efficiency
- Excellent skills for researching and tracking down information
- Understanding of what is of interest to funders
- Ability to construct an accurate budget plan
- Willingness to accept criticism and make changes

Compensation

According to a salary survey by the American Association of Grant Professionals, respondents with grant proposal writing as their primary responsibility earned an average of $54,717 in 2009. Many grant writers work as independent contractors and are paid by the hour or by the project; hourly rates may be as low as $30 or $40 or as high as $100 or more, depending on the writer's experience and credentials.

Workplaces

Grant writers with a public health focus work for nonprofits, academic research institutions, state or local agencies, and some private companies. Some write grant proposals for these types of organizations but do so as freelancers, which means they have their own offices or work from home and set their own hours.

Employment Outlook

Grants are what keep many public health programs running and allow innovative new programs to start, so there will always be a need for people with the skills to write grant applications. Getting started can be tricky without experience; volunteering in the fundraising department at a reputable organization can help.

For Further Information

- The Grantsmanship Center
  www.tgci.com
- The Foundation Center
  foundationcenter.org
- American Association of Grant Professionals (AAGP)
  grantprofessionals.org
- American Grant Writers Association
  www.agwa.us

DEVELOPMENT DIRECTOR

Job Description

Not-for-profit groups dedicated to public health can require a lot of work to keep themselves running, and that means finding money to support their day-to-day operations and services. The development director is the one who keeps the money coming in. He or she makes short-term and long-range plans for fundraising, coordinates efforts to carry out these plans, maintains relationships with funders, and looks for new ways to find support. Funders can include government agencies, other nonprofits, local or national corporations, and wealthy individuals. Depending on the size of the organization, development directors either do specific fundraising tasks themselves or oversee the people who do. This includes tracking down the right people, arranging meetings, explaining why a particular funder might want to support the organization, and writing grant proposals. When funding is received, they keep in touch with the funders and let them know how their money is being used. They also plan fundraising events and keep people aware of the organization, such as through writing newsletters or press releases. Development directors are usually outgoing, social people who enjoy interacting with funders and are not afraid to ask for what an organization needs. These jobs are based in comfortable, professional office settings but also include many outside meetings and often a number of evening or weekend fundraising events.

Education and Certification

There is no specific educational requirement for development directors, but a bachelor's degree is usually the minimum and a higher degree is common. Experience with grant writing or other fundraising, in a lower-level job or one with related responsibilities, is extremely helpful. Organizations usually look for people with connections in the area of public health they serve or with the proven ability to make such connections. For those who want to pursue specialized training, certificate programs are available at a number of universities. A Certified Fund Raising Executive (CFRE) credential can be helpful, although it not generally considered essential. (Details are at www.cfre.org.)

Core Competencies and Skills

- Outgoing personality
- Creative thinking
- Excellent communication skills
- Knack for seeing how funders' interests might coincide with those of the organization
- Good long-term planning skills
- Ability to meet deadlines
- Understanding of budgeting and of how fundraising works
- Passion for the work the organization does

Compensation

A salary survey by the American Association of Grant Professionals found that grant coordinators and fundraisers earned about $62,000 per year in 2009. The Association of Fundraising Professionals reports that among their members, chief development officers earned a median salary of $72,000; salaries were higher at state and national organizations, compared with local ones. For deputy development officers, the median salary was $62,000. Salaries can rise to $100,000 or above with extensive experience.

Workplaces

Development directors are typically found at nonprofit organizations and at other organizations, such as academic institutions, that rely on grants from outside funders.

Employment Outlook

Fundraising will always be an important part of the nonprofit world, and at any given moment there are multiple openings for development directors around the United States. However, people who want to get started in development work may need some flexibility. At smaller nonprofits people tend to wear many hats, and if there is a dedicated development department, it may have just one full-time employee.

For Further Information

- American Association of Fundraising Professionals (AFP)
  www.afpnet.org

PROGRAM OFFICER

Job Description

A program officer oversees grantmaking by a nonprofit foundation or a government agency, for a specific area of research or services. He or she is involved in deciding who should receive grants and how funding should be distributed. This includes planning a long-term strategy to meet the foundation's goals, keeping track of what has already been funded, and identifying areas where new work would be especially valuable. The program officer writes requests for proposals, outlining the type of projects the foundation or agency would like to support, and may also contact researchers directly to suggest projects. As grant proposals come in, the program officer evaluates them to decide which projects should receive funding. Once a grant has been given to an organization or researcher, the program officer keeps an eye on the recipient's work. He or she looks at periodic reports and may pay a visit to the laboratory or community site. The program officer reviews the progress of the project, checks to see if goals are being met, ensures that grant money is being spent appropriately, and recommends specific changes if needed. Program officers also connect with other organizations and speak to the public to promote the foundation's or agency's goals, and they attend research meetings and conferences to keep up with current trends.

In addition to program officers who focus on funding for research, there are also many people with this job title who handle funding for health promotion programs and other public health efforts.

Education and Certification

A bachelor's degree is the minimum requirement for a program officer job. A master's degree is often preferred and may be required. In some situations, the program officer must have a PhD or other terminal degree, because he or she needs a high-level of expertise to understand the proposed projects and make judgments about them; this is typical in the federal government. Relevant experience is usually required, and people with experience doing the type of work a foundation or agency funds will often have a competitive edge.

Core Competencies and Skills

- Tendency toward critical thinking and the ability to see how a project fits into larger goals
- Excellent verbal and written communication skills
- Confidence in public speaking and making presentations
- Ability to handle multiple projects at once
- At least a basic understanding of statistics and epidemiology
- Strong understanding of the field of work being funded, including current knowledge, needs, past successes and failures, and ongoing research and services
- Awareness of needs assessment methods, such as determining the true need for a proposed research study, or for community services in a specific location

■ Knowledge of regulations and requirements regarding grantmaking and nonprofit organizations

Compensation

Program officer salaries vary widely, depending on the complexity of the work, the funding available, and the experience and education required. According to the Council on Foundations, in 2008 the median salary for a program officer at a nonprofit was about $77,000; senior program officers can earn $100,000 per year or more.

Workplaces

Program officers work at nonprofit organizations and government agencies. Many large companies also sponsor foundations to manage their philanthropic goals.

Employment Outlook

There tends to be competition for program officer jobs, because many people find the idea of grantmaking appealing.

For Further Information

■ Council on Foundations
  www.cof.org
■ Grantmakers in Health (GIH)
  www.gih.org

PUBLIC HEALTH PROFILE: Program Officer
Brenda Henry, PhD, MPH
Research and Evaluation Program Officer
Robert Wood Johnson Foundation, Princeton, NJ

Describe the sort of work you do.

The Robert Wood Johnson Foundation (RWJF) gives grants to organizations that help us achieve our mission, which is about improving health and health care for all Americans. We fund programs that

Continued

improve health directly, programs that inform citizens and policymakers, and original research. The area I work in involves grants to support new research that helps fill in knowledge gaps, as well as grants to support program evaluation. My specific grant areas are public health and vulnerable populations.

What is a typical day like at your job?

My assistant keeps track of my calendar, so I start by looking to see what's scheduled. Then, I spend my day on a number of different tasks. There are calls with grantees to get status updates, find out what's going on with their programs, and talk about any issues. I read grant proposals, and I write new requests for proposals on topics our foundation is interested in. I do a lot of presentations at conferences, so on many days I work on creating slides and writing talks.

Our funding team meets regularly to decide which proposals to approve. I write and present summaries of the proposals I think should be funded. The other team members ask questions, and then they vote.

My job involves a fair amount of traveling. I often attend academic meetings to hear grantees present their findings. For the evaluation grants, I'll sometimes go to see the program that is being evaluated. I also go to conferences to get ideas and to see if there is something we might want to be involved in supporting.

What education or training do you have? Is it typical for your job?

I have a bachelor's in health science, an MPH, and a PhD in public health. Our program officers come from many disciplines and have different levels of education. You need to have the right education and experience to understand the grant proposals. A few of my colleagues are RNs or have other relevant degrees.

What path did you take to get to the job you are in today?

I worked for about 4 years with an academic research group, as a research assistant and then as program coordinator. But I wanted a

Continued

job that would let me take the research results and actually translate them into programs that would benefit the populations we were studying. So I went back to school for the MPH, and then on to earn the PhD. I worked at a small nonprofit for a couple years, helping organizations that ran programs for teens to improve their services. I wasn't looking to leave that job, but I met someone who was working at RWJF—and she suggested that with my interests, I might like to work there, too. I thought, "I won't lose anything by interviewing!" And it turned out that this job would give me a chance to have an even larger impact.

Where might you go from here, if you wanted to advance your career?

A lot of people make their whole careers being program officers, and it never gets boring because the work you're focusing on changes all the time. I do want to go back into academia eventually, but I'm not sure exactly when. If I decide I'd like to stay, the next step would be senior program officer, with more of a role in shaping initiatives. From there, one might move to deputy director, handling more of the administrative functioning, and then gain increasing responsibility from there.

What is the worst or most challenging part of your job?

I have to make hard decisions about what we are and aren't going to fund. We're a large foundation, but we have a finite amount of resources. The worst part is coming to terms with the fact that there might be something that I'm passionate about, but because it isn't in line with our strategic direction, we just can't support it.

What is the best part?

Everything that I do has the goal of making a positive impact on the health of Americans. I love every single aspect of my job! I also like the fact that I've been here for 2 years now and my job still challenges me in 101 different ways every day.

Continued

What advice do you have for someone who is interested in your career?

Hands-on work experience is essential. I wouldn't be good at this if I hadn't done what my grantees are doing, at some point. When I sit down and review a proposal, I have a sense of whether it is realistic, whether it can be done in the time frame suggested, and if the budget makes sense. There are questions I can ask that I wouldn't have known to ask if I hadn't done similar work.

VOLUNTEER COORDINATOR

Job Description

Nonprofit organizations that deal with public health issues tend to rely a lot on volunteers. But someone has to round up those volunteers, keep them organized, give them useful work to do, and ensure they follow any required regulations. That's what a volunteer coordinator does. Sometimes this person is a volunteer, too! But many organizations have someone on staff to do this job. An important part of the volunteer coordinator's work is attracting new volunteers. The coordinator keeps in touch with volunteers by phone or email, schedules projects for them to do, and oversees their efforts. The volunteer coordinator works with various departments at the organization to learn where volunteers are most needed and to find the most appropriate tasks for them to do. If volunteers must be trained or need to take certain classes, he or she arranges for this to happen. If something goes wrong—a volunteer makes a mistake, or someone gets upset—the coordinator steps in to handle the situation. Another part of the job is letting the volunteers know they are appreciated, with frequent thank-yous, small treats, and occasional special events. The volunteer coordinator might also write a newsletter, set up training workshops for volunteers, and pursue quality improvement efforts. This job combines deskwork with attendance at events where volunteers are needed and visits to locations, such as clinics or outreach centers, where volunteers are used.

Education and Certification

No special education or certification is required to become a volunteer coordinator, although most organizations will want someone with a bachelor's degree and/or supervisory experience. Volunteer administrators with a few years experience can choose to earn a Certified in Volunteer Administration credential from the Council for Certification in Volunteer Administration.

Core Competencies and Skills

- Patience
- Empathy
- Flexible thinking
- Good management skills
- High degree of comfort with meeting new people
- Dedication to and understanding of the organization's work
- Appreciation for the special role of volunteers, including an understanding of how expectations differ for volunteers and employees

Compensation

Salaries for volunteer coordinators tend to be modest. The Abbott, Langer Salary Survey for nonprofits suggests a median of $63,000 in 2007 for the title of "volunteer services director," but salaries for volunteer coordinators are often lower. The Web site salary.com, which offers information based on human resources data, gives a median salary of $39,000 in 2009, with most earning $30,000 to $53,000.

Workplaces

Volunteer coordinators whose work addresses public health issues often work for nonprofit organizations. Some health departments and other government agencies have volunteer coordinators, too. They may have duties similar to those at a nonprofit, enlisting volunteers to help with public health campaigns and community programs. Some manage a reserve corps of health care professionals and other skilled workers who have agreed to help in case of a public health emergency; this job involves more administrative and program management tasks.

Employment Outlook

Finding a paid volunteer coordinator job requires patience and a bit of luck. Sometimes this position is combined with another one, so that the office manager or program director might also manage the volunteers. Sometimes it is a part-time job. Job stability depends on available funding.

For Further Information

■ Volunteering in America
www.volunteeringinamerica.gov
■ Association of Leaders in Volunteer Engagement (AL!VE)
www.volunteeralive.org

DIRECTOR OF A PROFESSIONAL ASSOCIATION

Job Description

Professional associations are not-for-profit organizations with members comprising physicians, nurses, or other health care or public health professionals. They focus on one aspect of medicine or public health and serve to educate the public, set guidelines, give members opportunities for networking and education, and advocate for public health issues. These organizations have boards of directors consisting of members who have been elected to help guide the organization. But they also employ executives to lead and manage the organization on the administrative side. These top managers have various titles, such as CEO, Executive Director, or President; they are different from the elected Chair or President, who serves for a year at a time. The Executive Director is, essentially, the business manager. He or she focuses on the nuts and bolts of improving membership, arranging partnerships with other organizations, finding funding, communicating with local chapters, keeping the Web site useful and organized, making sure that the association keeps to its annual budget, and ensuring that the association remains influential and viable over the long-term. Depending on the size of the association, he or she may oversee a small number of employees or a large staff. The job includes making and maintaining connections with political leaders and other influential people and serving as a spokesperson for the association. The Executive Director also offers recommendations to the elected board members and works with them to further the association's objectives.

Education and Certification

There is no set pathway to becoming the chief executive at a professional association. Some organizations prefer people with degrees related to the association's work, such as an MD, DO, or MPH. Others look for people with administrative experience. Experience managing an organization or department is key. Some administrators choose to pursue the Certified Association Executive (CAE) credential, which requires several years of experience in association management, relevant continuing education, and an examination.

Core Competencies and Skills

- Superb organizational skills
- Excellent leadership and strategic planning skills
- Ability to manage a large number of projects at once
- Ability to remain calm under pressure
- Confidence in the face of differing opinions
- Strong skills in business, such as financial management and negotiation
- Deep understanding of the association's focus and of important issues in that field, including health, economic, and legislative issues

Compensation

Salaries for the directors of professional societies have an extremely wide-range. The executive director at one of the smaller professional associations takes home a base salary of about $125,000 each year; another, in a state where the cost of living is lower, around $70,000. At the high end is a top administrator at a major national medical association, who earns well over half a million dollars each year.

Workplaces

This job is found at nonprofit professional societies and similar associations, such as coalitions of community organizations.

Employment Outlook

Top positions at major national organization require extensive experience, but smaller associations will sometimes be open to hiring someone with the right credentials but a limited track record. There are also many other opportunities to participate in running a nonprofit organization, including a professional society, at entry- and mid-level positions.

For Further Information

■ American Society of Association Executives (ASAE)
www.asaecenter.org

PUBLIC HEALTH PROFILE: Director of a Professional Association
Mike Barry
Executive Director
American College of Preventive Medicine (ACPM), Washington, DC

Describe the sort of work you do.

ACPM is a professional medical society for physicians in preventive medicine. Our members occupy a unique niche at the intersection between clinical medicine and public health. ACPM's mission is two-fold: to serve as the leader of the speciality of preventive medicine, and to work toward the broader goal of improving population health. As executive director, I'm responsible for carrying out the strategic plan set by our board of directors. I oversee operations, finance, business development, and the whole array of activities that are carried out by the College. That includes managing internal functions such as our annual conference and membership support, and also forging partnerships with aligned external corporations, nonprofits, and government agencies to develop new ways to promote better health. Those partnerships increase our visibility, expand our capacity, and provide revenue to keep the organization running.

What is a typical day like at your job?

On any given day, I usually have several meetings and teleconferences dealing with the range of activities in which the organization is involved: for example, meeting with potential partners, talking with our development officer about raising funds, or holding teleconferences with our Board or committees about what they want to accomplish. I spend a lot of time on email and meeting directly with staff. I also review a lot of documents—anything with ACPM's name on it.

One important part of my job is deciding what projects and partnerships we should pursue. For example, ACPM has been working with a government agency on increasing awareness about the implications of

Continued

climate change for public health, and we recently submitted a grant proposal to advance the effort further. Preparing a grant proposal is a lot of work, and I had to decide whether the opportunity looked promising enough to justify my staff's time and effort. I also provide guidance on shaping projects to best fit our capabilities and our mission, and I'm involved regularly in negotiating contracts. At the moment, we're renegotiating a contract with a company that uses some of our educational tools.

What education or training do you have? Is it typical for your job?

I have a bachelor's degree in mathematics and a CAE credential. Different organizations have different requirements. Some boards want their executive director to have the same credentials that members have. In its most recent search, ACPM decided that my experience with professional associations and background in public health matched their needs.

What path did you take to get to the job you are in today?

When I started my career, I had no aspirations to work in public health or associations. I wanted a job that dealt with statistics and data analysis. I responded to an ad for a statistical assistant at an organization called the Public Health Foundation and discovered that I really liked the nonprofit world and doing research, policy, and other kinds of work around public health. I stayed with that organization for 14 years, learned to do project management, and eventually rose to the level of senior director. And then the executive director of ACPM, who earlier had been the deputy director at the Public Health Foundation, recruited me. I was deputy director here for 5 years, and when the executive director stepped down, I threw my hat in the ring.

Where might you go from here, if you wanted to advance your career?

I haven't thought much about life after ACPM. I like what I'm doing. I think with the path I've taken, I could move on to any other association in the same role. Or, if I decided I didn't want to be the chief executive

Continued

anymore, I could take on a lower-level senior position in a larger organization, one with more divisions and staff and a higher budget.

What is the worst or most challenging part of your job?

The decisions I make every day affect the success of the organization. That can bring a lot of stress! One of the most difficult things about my job is that we are a small organization with limited financial resources, and the world of preventive medicine is so broad. So we have to say no to some opportunities, and sometimes we can't do what the board or president wants to do. I have to find other ways to approach those goals.

What is the best part?

No two days are alike. I'm never bored. The job fits my personality well, because it is a generalist job. I deal with the entire gamut of the organization but do not get mired in the technical aspects.

What advice do you have for someone who is interested in your career?

I don't know of anyone in this field (running nonprofit associations) who planned it as a career. Most people start at a nonprofit because they are interested in the cause. Once you realize you are good at it and you enjoy it, you naturally work your way up the ladder. If you aspire to be a senior director or chief staff executive, learn everything you can about all aspects of the organization. Talk to colleagues, learn what they do, pay attention at staff meetings. The more you understand the big picture, the more ready you'll be to assume a leadership position.

20 Public Health Administration and Leadership

There are several careers in earlier chapters that could fall into the category of "administration and leadership," and many of the others can be steps on the way to a leadership position. This chapter offers a special focus on the jobs that help shape public health efforts at local, state, and national levels.

All of these roles require significant leadership skills. Some are more administrative; some are more in the public eye. They all share a need for excellent strategic planning skills, with the ability to see the "big picture" both for the immediate moment and for years down the road.

In most cases, these are not jobs you'll apply for straight out of school. They're jobs you grow into. There are a number of programs designed to help shape future public health leaders. There are training opportunities at the CDC, there is a list of leadership programs at the Public Health Leadership Society (phls.org), and an Internet search for "public health leadership institutes" will also bring up opportunities. There is also an APHA section for Health Administration (www.apha.org).

To learn more about jobs where leadership is a primary focus, revisit director/emergency medical services, deputy director/family health services, director/state board of pharmacy, and dean/school of public health, and see the Public Health Profile for medical officer/drug safety. Strong leadership and administration skills are also particularly important for corporate medical director, director/office of minority health, president and CEO/area agency on aging, director of a professional organization, and nongovernmental organization founder/director.

HEALTH COMMISSIONER

Job Description

"Commissioner" is a title used for the head of a health department, with "deputy commissioners" overseeing specific areas within the department. (Not all health departments use these titles; the top person may be called "Director" or "Secretary of Health.") The commissioner has the final word on many decisions about future directions, major programs, and how the budget is managed. He or she decides where and how resources should be used and what health issues should be addressed. When an important choice must be made, such as whether to close the schools to combat a flu outbreak, the commissioner takes responsibility. He or she advocates for the department with city, county, or state government and makes sure that the department has the budget, personnel, legal and policy framework, and overall capability to respond to the city, county, or state's public health needs, now and in the future. The commissioner also represents the department in conversations with media, legislators, leaders of other health agencies, health care providers, and other stakeholders.

Health departments often have deputy commissioners to manage sections of the department. Under the direction of the commissioner, they develop short- and long-term goals for specific areas of public health, set priorities, and play key roles in policy development. They manage decisions about spending within their areas of responsibility. Other tasks include leading quality improvement efforts, supervising staff, and collaborating with other agencies and community groups.

Education and Certification

Some jurisdictions require the health commissioner to be a licensed physician; there are also commissioners who are nurses, who have MPH degrees, or who have other credentials. Many physician commissioners also have an MPH or an MPA, and some have MBAs or JDs. Similarly, deputy commissioners may be MDs or DOs or may have other training, depending on local requirements. It is typical to have prior experience within the health department or as administrator in another health-oriented agency or organization.

Core Competencies and Skills

- Excellent management skills
- Ability to juggle multiple projects at once
- Good political skills and understanding of local politics
- Patience with bureaucracy and red tape
- Ability to remain calm under pressure
- Excellent public speaking skills
- Understanding of epidemiology and of the principles of public health
- Knowledge of the public health infrastructure at both local and national levels
- Knowledge of local, state, and national health issues, programs, laws, and regulations

Compensation

Health commissioners earn comfortable salaries. Typical salaries range from about $90,000 per year in a mid-western county to nearly $200,000 in a major eastern city. Deputy commissioners are generally paid less than the top executive.

Workplaces

Health commissioners and deputy commissioners (or executives with similar jobs but different titles) lead health departments at the city, county, and state levels.

Employment Outlook

The top jobs go to people who have substantial administrative and leadership experience and are well respected in the local community or in the field of public health. In some cities and counties, there are opportunities for physicians and others with appropriate training, but without extensive administrative experience, to obtain assistant or deputy commissioner jobs. Most top state and territorial health officials and many local commissioners or directors are political appointees, so elections can affect job stability.

For Further Information

- National Association of City and County Health Officials (NACCHO) *www.naccho.org*
- Association of State and Territorial Health Officials (ASTHO) *www.astho.org*

PUBLIC HEALTH PROFILE: Deputy Health Commissioner
Teré Dickson, MD, MPH

Deputy Commissioner of Health, Director of the Center for Social Health and Advocacy
Nassau County Department of Health, Uniondale, NY

Describe the sort of work you do.

As a deputy commissioner, my official role is to assist the county health commissioner in advancing the mission of the health department, which is to "protect, promote, and prevent." I have several specific responsibilities. I oversee the bureaus of HIV, sexually transmitted disease, and tuberculosis. I am in charge of HIV prevention and outreach, and I manage our health disparities grants. I advocate for the health needs of minority communities in ways that will address health disparities. And I act as community liaison to minority groups, as well as to the county legislature.

What is a typical day like at your job?

I usually start my day with tasks related to payroll. Then I'll answer emails from people like the commissioner, community representatives, my staff, and staff from other agencies. I often have a couple of meetings in the morning. There may be a staff meeting, or an update about a disease outbreak. I might meet with community-based organizations, and sometimes we invite individual community residents to share their thoughts with us. We also meet with hospitals to discuss potential collaborations.

Continued

In the afternoon, I'll have a couple hours to handle any writing I have to do, such as a grant proposal, a monthly report to the Board of Health, or talking points for the head of our county government. Sometimes I work on presentations for the commissioner to use. I prepare my own presentations to give at schools, community groups, and government programs. Sometimes I'll have grant reports to review and approve. I also use my afternoons to return phone calls and respond to requests for information. Some evenings I'll have an additional meeting.

What education or training do you have? Is it typical for your job?

I have an MD and an MPH. You have to have a professional degree to hold a job at this level. Some counties will have a director who is a nurse, but county commissioners and deputy commissioners tend to have medical degrees. For my position the county wanted someone with both a medical degree and an MPH, but it is common for our commissioners not to have an MPH. Sometimes one will have an MPA.

What path did you take to get to the job you are in today?

I volunteered at a hospital during college, and just being in that environment was very energizing. But then I got to medical school and my pediatrics residency, and I found that my patients were struggling with problems that, as a clinical physician, I had no control over. The turning point was a teenage girl, 15 years old, who came to me for a checkup. She had multiple sexual partners in the past year —and when I mentioned birth control, she didn't know what that was. She was from an ethnic minority group, and it made me wonder—this information is out there in abundance, how come it hadn't reached this girl? I started thinking about health communication and how it could be used to address these kinds of problems in minority populations.

I went on to do a second residency, this time in preventive medicine. During that time I worked at a county office of minority health, and that helped me see how to get things done. I also spent some

Continued

time at a news organization and working on health media and marketing projects, so I learned more about communicating health information. Around the time I graduated, Nassau County was looking for a deputy commissioner with an interest in health disparities, and they liked the set of skills that I had.

Where might you go from here, if you wanted to advance your career?

In a health department, one potential career ladder is to go from medical supervisor to division director, then to deputy commissioner, and then, if the job is available, to commissioner. For myself, though, one possibility I'm considering is to create a consulting service for health disparities programming and communications. I also like the idea of working as a media doctor or medical correspondent, using television, radio, print, and the Internet to educate people and help them make better choices about their health.

What is the worst or most challenging part of your job?

Personnel management can be tough. There is a lot of office politics, too. As someone relatively new to the department, I've had to find my way through that.

What is the best part?

I like doing community presentations. It is the only communications piece that I get to do right now, and it gives me a chance to be creative. I like interacting with people, learning their mindset, and getting a sense of the knowledge level in the communities. I especially like talking to kids—they have fun questions.

What advice do you have for someone who is interested in your career?

Get as much experience as you can before you become the boss. Look at people who are successful, and observe and try to understand the communication and time management skills they use. Test the waters while it's not crucial—try to spend some time at the health department during residency, for example. Make sure to learn about the work before you're in a position to be held accountable for it.

PUBLIC HEALTH LABORATORY DIRECTOR

Job Description

Public health laboratories are different from hospital laboratories. They are charged with helping to protect everyone's health and safety. They diagnose and monitor infectious diseases and other health threats, screen for genetic problems in newborns, and do certain types of environmental testing. They have the knowledge and capability to watch for bioterrorism agents, too. Certain complex or unusual tests, such as rabies and smallpox, are done only at public health labs. (The actual scope and quantity of testing differs from place to place according to local needs.) A public health laboratory director leads diagnostics and monitoring within his or her jurisdiction and serves as the point person for coordination of laboratory response when there is a public health crisis. Together with other public health and health care leaders, the director develops plans to meet current and future needs, so that the laboratory can provide essential services as completely and efficiently as possible. He or she advocates for funding and resources to maintain a state-of-the-art facility with the capacity to do all necessary testing. The director keeps an eye on the quality of work at the laboratory, designing and implementing quality improvement systems and also overseeing employee schedules, equipment maintenance, disease reporting, and compliance with federal regulations.

Education and Certification

In most jurisdictions, a public health laboratory director must have a PhD in a field related to chemical, physical, biological or clinical laboratory science, or an MD or DO degree plus pathology board certification or related experience. PhDs must also be certified by one of several boards approved by HHS. Individual states have their own specific requirements, such as a state license or certification.

Core Competencies and Skills

- Strong administrative and management skills, for oversight of budgeting, personnel, and equipment
- Good public relations and public speaking skills
- Knowledge of grant writing and business development
- Experience with quality monitoring and improvement

- Knowledge of public health principles and of the public health infrastructure
- Expertise in microbiology, bacteriology, biochemistry, or a related discipline
- Up-to-date knowledge of testing methods used in health care and environmental monitoring
- Understanding of federal regulations and requirements for laboratory work

Compensation

The salary for a public health laboratory director depends on the size of the laboratory, the population it serves, and the department budget. In a 2007/2008 survey published by *ADVANCE*, a magazine for laboratory professionals, the average salary for a laboratory's administrative director was $74,690; the survey included public health labs but did not report that data separately. Some recent examples for public health laboratory directors include county salaries of about $60,000 to $100,000 in a Western state, $65,000 to $94,000 for a state laboratory director in the Midwest, and $120,000 for a state laboratory director in a Northeastern state.

Workplaces

Public health laboratory directors serve at all levels of government, usually working within health agencies.

Employment Outlook

Public health laboratory scientists are great demand, and there should be increasing opportunities as current public health laboratory workers retire over the next decade. There is also a strong need for other laboratory scientists, from entry level technicians to laboratory managers and senior scientists with masters' and doctoral degrees.

For Further Information

- Association of Public Health Laboratories (APHL)
  www.aphl.org

■ LabAspire
www.labaspire.org

MEDICAL DIRECTOR

Job Description

"Medical Director" is a title that can refer to a lot of different jobs. Throughout public health settings, medical directors are physicians who contribute their specialized knowledge to the development and implementation of services and programs. A medical director at a health department provides medical expertise regarding the many health care and health policy issues that arise. He or she serves as the liaison with outside clinical professionals and professional associations. He or she may also oversee the department's clinical services and even provide direct patient care. Public health agencies may also have medical directors in more specific roles. For example, a city health department's bureau of emergency management might have a medical director to guide planning for the medical response to a disaster. In an EMS system, a physician keeps an eye on the training of emergency medical technicians and paramedics and makes decisions about care protocols, so that the services provided are consistent with the latest medical knowledge. Departments of corrections have medical directors to ensure that inmates receive quality care that not only protects their health, but also helps protect the health of the community after they are released.

Education and Certification

A medical director must be a licensed physician with training and experience appropriate to the role. A job may require experience in medical practice, supervisory experience, public health experience, or some combination of these. An MPH or board certification in public health and general preventive medicine can be an advantage.

Core Competencies and Skills

- Strong management skills
- Excellent written and verbal communication skills
- High degree of comfort with public speaking

- Ability to work with both medical and nonclinical personnel and to explain medical concepts in plain English
- Good understanding of epidemiology, statistics, and how to read surveillance reports and research studies
- Strong knowledge of clinical medicine, particularly of issues that are commonly addressed by public health efforts
- Thorough understanding of public health techniques and principles
- At least a basic understanding of the public health system and of public health law

Compensation

Medical directors' salaries are fairly typical for physicians, although generally closer to a primary care doctor's salary than to that of a highly paid specialist. A range of $100,000 to $200,000 is common, although jobs may pay less or more depending on budget, experience, and level of responsibility. Recent examples include about $130,000 for a medical director in an emergency preparedness program in a major Midwestern city and well over $200,000 for the top medical director job at a county health department in a large metropolitan area.

Workplaces

There are medical directors at local and state health departments. When public health services are divided among other local or state agencies, these agencies may also employ medical directors. Nonprofit organizations that provide services often have medical directors, as well.

Employment Outlook

An anticipated shortage of public health physicians suggests that there will be an ongoing need for qualified people to serve as medical directors. At the same time, the number of these jobs within each health agency is limited.

For Further Information

- See the organizations listed with health commissioner.

FEDERAL AGENCY DIRECTOR

Job Description

The CDC has a top director to guide the agency's work, and each of its many divisions also has a director who shapes that division's agenda. Other federal agencies dealing with the public's health, such as the FDA, have similar structures, although the titles may be different. Directors can have enormous influence, serving as nationally and internationally recognized experts. They provide leadership on public health issues and encourage research on disease prevention and health promotion. They develop and maintain relationships with other federal agencies, state and local health departments, academic institutions, and national organizations. They are involved in creating health policy, carrying out new policies, and maximizing the efficiency and effectiveness of the department. Although they delegate much of the day-to-day administrative work, they bear responsibility for all major activities within the agency, from financial matters to decisions about drug approvals or health initiatives. They also have the privilege of providing direction and vision to the agency on a wide range of public health issues.

Education and Certification

Becoming the director of a federal public health agency, or of a division within such an agency, requires a doctoral degree in a related field and a strong track record in public health work. Many people start out in lower-level jobs at local health departments or at federal agencies, and then work up through the ranks. The current CDC Director, for example, worked with the CDC for many years before becoming Commissioner of the New York City Health Department. From there, he was tapped for his current job.

Core Competencies and Skills

- High degree of expertise in public health, with specific expertise related to the agency's work
- High degree of prominence in the world of public health
- Experience in public health leadership, program development, and program implementation
- Experience with government, academia, and health-related

organizations, to allow effective communication and collaboration
- Experience interacting with reporters and the public

Compensation

Leaders in the federal government are well compensated, although often not as well as people with similar levels of responsibility in the private business world. For example, in 2008, the Director of the CDC earned a base salary of $172,000, according to a federal salary database, and the FDA Commissioner earned $191,300.

Employment Outlook

As with other leadership jobs, there are only a few top positions, and they are open only to people with proven leadership skills and a high level of accomplishment. There are many lower-level leadership opportunities, however, which can lead eventually to positions of greater influence.

For Further Information

- To learn more about how federal agencies such as the CDC are run, visit their Web sites and look for links labeled "about" or "organization."

SURGEON GENERAL OF THE UNITED STATES

Job Description

Known as America's Doctor, the Surgeon General is responsible for helping Americans understand how to improve their health and reduce their risk of illness and injury. The Surgeon General's duties include educating the public, advocating for effective public health programs, and serving as a symbol of the nation's commitment to protecting and improving our citizens' health. Through the Office of the Surgeon General, he or she oversees the U.S. Public Health Service Commissioned Corps. The Surgeon General advises the President, the Secretary of Health and Human Services, and other government officials on a wide range of health issues, based on the best scientific evidence and policy analysis. He or she works with other agencies to promote specific initiatives, such as preventing HIV prevention or reducing obesity. Responsibilities also include raising the standards for and quality of public health practice, promoting essential research, and contributing to emergency preparedness planning. The Surgeon General oversees the publication of major reports on health issues, convenes workshops with key leaders in public health, encourages community programs, and speaks out in the media about priority issues. In many ways, each Surgeon General is able to decide how to shape the job and how best to use the public influence it offers.

Education and Certification

The Surgeon General must be a physician and is typically an accomplished public health leader.

Core Competencies and Skills

- Passion for public health
- Understanding of public health issues on both the local and national scales
- Excellent management and interpersonal skills
- Ability to juggle multiple projects while keeping up with a busy schedule
- High level of comfort with public speaking, including media appearances
- Ability to select issues that can and should be addressed on a national scale
- Understanding of the use of evidence-based practice
- Ability to mobilize public health leaders and the public to take effective action

Compensation

The surgeon general's salary is about $150,000.

Employment Outlook

There is only one U.S. Surgeon General. It is not the sort of job you can apply for. The President selects someone to hold this post, and only the most accomplished physicians are considered. The doctor President

Obama chose in 2009 was "just" a family physician who ran a clinic in a rural area of Alabama—but she also had a long list of achievements and awards. She had been chair of the Federation of State Medical Boards of the United States, president of the American Medical Association Education and Research Foundation, and associate dean at a medical school. She had served on many influential boards and committees and been recognized, multiple times, for her accomplishments.

For Further Information

- Office of the Surgeon General
  www.surgeongeneral.gov

21 Global Health

Defining "global public health" is a bit of a challenge. A recent commentary in *The Lancet* offers the perspective that global health *is* public health, with a shared emphasis on population-level policies, health promotion, and health as a broad concept encompassing physical, mental, and social well-being. Further, attention to health around the world is important for controlling infectious disease transmission, sharing information about preventing or ameliorating chronic diseases, and creating the most efficient and effective systems for the delivery of health care.

A look at courses and departments at American schools of public health reveals a wide range of "global health" work attached to public health research, education, and practice. There are programs focused on HIV prevention, infant nutrition, water and sanitation, the control of malaria, family planning, and many more areas of health. There are programs to build or strengthen the public health infrastructure. There are projects examining health disparities, studying ways to prevent violence, addressing health impacts of globalization, and more.

Some of the other jobs and careers in this book are closely linked with global health. Most of the careers in the Infectious Disease chapter and several in the Chronic Disease chapter include connections with global health. There are jobs with global health elements for pharmacists, biostatisticians, environmental engineers, nutrition consultants, consumer safety officers, emergency preparedness specialists, social marketers, professors, program evaluators, and many others. Evaluation is a particularly hot topic in global health right now.

There are many nonprofits, government agencies, and intergovernmental organizations concerned with global health. Here are a few places to start:

- The APHA section on International Health (www.apha.org/ membergroups/sections/aphasections)
- The Global Fund (theglobalfund.org)
- World Health Organization (www.who.int)
- UNAIDS (www.unaids.org)
- UNICEF (www.unicef.org)
- CDC Global Health (www.cdc.gov/globalhealth)
- USAID (www.usaid.gov)
- The Gates Foundation (www.gatesfoundation.org)

PHYSICIAN/GLOBAL HEALTH

Job Description

Doctors have many opportunities to shape public health programs in the developing world, serving as advisors or working directly in research, systems and program design, and evaluation. For example, there are doctors involved in building capacity for HIV prevention and treatment in countries in Africa. They help decide what training local health care providers need and contribute to the design and implementation of that training. They travel to clinics to make sure they are properly staffed and that they have the necessary space and equipment. Physicians are also involved in decreasing the impact of other chronic or infectious diseases, designing mental health services, and many other aspects of public health in the developing world. They may be based in the United States and travel to other countries periodically, or be based overseas.

Education and Certification

A medical degree is essential. Each job has its own requirements, depending on the work to be done. Some physicians who do international public health work specialize in tropical medicine. Some are preventive medicine specialists. Some have other specialties plus training in public health. Employers look for doctors with skills and training that match a particular program or population's needs. They also look for people with experience living and working abroad, ideally in the region where the work will be focused.

Core Competencies and Skills

- Adaptability
- Interest in other cultures and awareness of local climate, customs, and politics
- Fluency in a relevant language or the ability to learn (helpful and sometimes essential)
- Strong knowledge of epidemiology
- Expertise in the field of work to be done
- Understanding of the local health care capabilities and how they differ from what is available in the United States.

Compensation

Salaries differ according to agency, duty location, and specific job. Here are some recent examples. A WHO medical officer assigned to help with yellow fever control in Africa, with at least several years experience in this type of work, could earn about $106,000. A CDC medical officer helping with HIV prevention and control, based in the United States and traveling overseas, could earn $85,000 to $111,000.

Workplaces

The WHO, the USAID, and the CDC all employ medical officers to do global health work. Physicians can work for consulting firms that contract with international health agencies. There are also many nonprofit organizations that employ physicians to help with global health efforts, and there are opportunities for international public health work in the military. The U.S. Public Health Service Commissioned Corps is another option.

Employment Outlook

In 2009, the CDC was actively recruiting for medical officers with skills in epidemiology to work overseas. Other job titles to look for are "technical officer" and "health scientist," which often require an MD or PhD.

Getting started can be a challenge, because many jobs are for people with experience, but seeking international health internships and fellowships and taking advantage of volunteer opportunities can lead to a first international job. Once established, international public health experts often enjoy long and interesting careers.

For Further Information

There are too many organizations concerned with global health and prevention to list them all here. There is a useful introduction to CDC career opportunities at:

- CDC Global Health—Jobs Overseas
  www.cdc.gov/globalhealth/employment.htm

TECHNICAL ADVISOR/LOGISTICS

Job Description

Technical advisors share knowledge about how to make a system or a program work, with the goal of building a country's own capacity to do the work on its own; there are technical advisors with expertise in many areas, from maternal and child health to water and sanitation. A technical advisor with expertise in logistics focuses on helping local governments or nongovernmental organizations (NGOs) forecast their supply needs and prepare to meet them. Take vaccines for example: Tracking the past year's use of vaccines, looking at plans to expand an immunization program, and figuring out how many vials, syringes, and alcohol wipes will be needed is a logistics job. The vaccines must be stored, shipped, and distributed in the right amounts to the right places; that's a logistics issue, too. Does the country have the capacity—transportation, storage space, communication networks, tracking programs, and workers—to handle a huge supply of vaccines all at once? If not, how can the system be improved, streamlined, or expanded? Will current funds be enough to purchase and deliver supplies, and if not, how can the program trim spending or obtain more funding? Logisticians also manage the flow of information and products so that vaccines don't expire before they are used, don't run out, and don't wind up sitting in a warehouse in one city, while a clinic in another region has none to distribute.

Education and Certification

The most common educational background for a logistician is a bachelor's degree, but this includes logisticians who work in business and industry, handling manufacturing supplies. Logistics experts in global health need more specialized knowledge and are often expected to have a master's degree, such as an MPH. A pharmacy degree, an MD, or a master's in business or logistics is also appropriate for some jobs.

Core Competencies and Skills

- Excellent teaching and communication skills
- Ability to work both independently and as part of a team
- Language skills or the ability—and patience—to work with translators
- Adaptability and a love of travel
- Strong customer service orientation
- Understanding of politics and the diplomatic ability to facilitate a discussion, negotiate delicate issues, and bring people to consensus
- Strong analytical and problem-solving skills, including the ability to extract key points from a large amount of information
- Tendency to be detail-oriented, combined with the ability to see the "big picture"
- Understanding of public health issues, with the ability to learn quickly about new topics and recognize the major issues

Compensation

In 2008, the median salary for a logistician was about $66,000 with most earning between $39,000 and $102,000. Technical advisors in logistics with 5 to 10 years of experience typically earn between $70,000 and $126,000.

Workplaces

Logistics experts, including technical advisors, work at international health and aid organizations and at consulting firms that contract with U.S. and international agencies and foundations. Organizations concerned with relief efforts following disasters also employ logistics experts; this work often has a public health element.

Employment Outlook

U.S. News and World Report lists logistician as one of the top 50 jobs for 2009, and the Bureau of Labor Statistics says jobs will increase rapidly—but they're primarily talking about the business world. This is a fairly small, specialized area in public health. There have been efforts over the past decade to strengthen supply chains in developing countries, with funding for technical advisors; the levels of continued interest, funding, and need will determine the number of future jobs for logistics experts.

For Further Information

- USAID DELIVER PROJECT
  deliver.jsi.com
- International Association of Public Health Logisticians (IAPHL)
  my.ibpinitiative.org
- Chartered Institute of Logistics and Transport
  www.cilt-international.com
- Fritz Institute
  www.fritzinstitute.org

PROCUREMENT MANAGER

Job Description

Most international public health programs require supplies. It could be posters and handouts for a social marketing campaign, or it could be clean syringes for a vaccination program. The procurement manager handles the purchasing of those items. But it is not as simple as just placing an order! Procuring enough supplies for a regional or nationwide program takes time, and it takes planning. The procurement manager helps program directors plan far in advance, to allow for manufacturing, shipping, clearance through customs, and distribution. He or she works with them to decide how to get the most for their money without compromising on quality or time, and ensures that the product will meet the program's needs. Then he or she gives manufacturers the requirements and timeline, obtains price quotes, and advises on any changes to the budget. After placing the order, the procurement manager keeps track of progress, arranges for quality testing, and reviews the results. The procurement manager plans in advance for shipping, considering everything from the method of transportation to problems that might arise at customs, and then monitors the shipment to make sure it arrives safely at its destination.

Education and Certification

A bachelor's degree in business, public administration, marketing, or a related field is a good place to start. An MPH can be helpful, too. Special training in procurement and contracts management is available through certificate programs at some universities. For those with experience who want professional certification, there is a Certified Professional in Supply Management credential available from the Institute for Supply Management.

Core Competencies and Skills

- Excellent organizational and planning skills especially for working within bureaucratic organizations
- High degree of common sense
- Good negotiating skills
- Good math skills and financial sense
- Ability to gather information effectively and determine what is important
- Understanding of how to differentiate between theory and practice
- Knack for explaining needs clearly, so that manufacturers know what is expected
- Ability to read and understand contracts
- Willingness to learn and gain experience over time

Compensation

The Institute of Supply Management's 2009 salary survey found an average of $47,869 for an entry-level supply management professional, to $93,132 for a Purchasing/Supply Management/Sourcing Manager, all the way up to $256,560 for the highest title. The average for people with 11 to 20 years of experience was $96,126.

Workplaces

There are opportunities available at consulting firms that contract with international agencies, nonprofits, and foreign governments, as well as at agencies and organizations that manage large public health programs.

Employment Outlook

There are not a lot of people with the specific skills and knowledge to do this type of work. After the entry level, opportunities should be good for someone who is willing to take the time and make the effort to gain experience.

For Further Information

- International Federation of Purchasing and Supply Management (IFPSM) *www.ifpsm.org*
- Council of Supply Chain Management Professionals (CSCMP) *cscmp.org*

PUBLIC HEALTH PROFILE: Procurement Manager
Paul Stannard
Deputy Procurement Manager
Crown Agents, Based at John Snow Inc., Arlington, VA

Describe the sort of work you do.

I'm currently assigned to work with John Snow, Inc., where I supervise a procurement team and also do a lot of the hands-on work myself. We procure products for international public health programs supported by USAID. That includes pharmaceuticals, medical devices, contraceptives, diagnostic tests, mosquito nets, and more. Purchases are informed by the receiving country's needs, what other donors are funding, and that country's own budget. My team and I work with the stakeholder in-country to figure out what to buy, how much to buy, and when. Then we handle purchasing, quality assurance, and shipping. If the country doesn't have the capacity to handle in country-transport, we'll arrange that too, all the way to local clinics or even individual households.

Continued

What is a typical day like at your job?

I'm in frequent contact with our field offices and U.S. embassies overseas, talking about requirements. For example, I'll talk with someone in Senegal about what supplies they need for their malaria control program. I speak regularly with manufacturers to negotiate terms, follow up on orders, and see if they are on schedule. Sometimes I'll be calling a manufacturer with an emergency order.

I also speak daily with my counterparts at USAID in Washington. Sometimes we need to discuss budget problems. Often, someone from USAID will call and ask my advice. I also keep in touch with our quality assurance experts about policies and practices, such as whether we need to sample more of a given product or can sample less.

About twice a year, I travel overseas. I go for a week or 10 days at a time. I do briefings for our field offices, explaining what we are doing, how we do it, and what they need to know. I also visit manufacturers' production facilities to discuss what we expect and what quality standards they need to meet.

What education or training do you have? Is it typical for your job?

I went to high school in the United Kingdom, and my higher exams were in the sciences. A lot of my colleagues have bachelor's degrees, which is expected for new people coming in. Many either have an MPH or are in the process of earning one. Very few have specific degrees related to procurement.

What path did you take to get to the job you are in today?

My original plan was to be a dentist. I took a year off after high school, and I wanted to travel. My careers advisor recommended that I get some work experience, and I was fortunate enough to join Crown Agents. I started in their shipping department. I got to go to Lagos when I was just 21. I spent a total of about a year and a half there, came home to England for a couple years, and then was sent to be a company representative in Singapore. My public health involvement started after that, when I helped set up a program to manage

Continued

essential drug procurement and distribution in Kenya. I spent a number of years running procurement projects and working in different African countries, and finally, as my last assignment came to an end, my wife and I decided to settle back in the United Kingdom. But then I was offered this posting in the United States, and here we are!

Where might you go from here, if you wanted to advance your career?

My plan for the future is to continue with supply chain work, whether directing a team, educating others, or consulting. It's difficult to describe a typical career progression, because structures differ from place to place. You start in a role with a lower amount of responsibility and as you learn, you gain more responsibility—but each job is different, so you never stop learning.

What is the worst or most challenging part of your job?

Sometimes our own donor bureaucracy or the bureaucracy in-country delays things, or the people in charge will make decisions that don't seem to make sense. It's also hard when people don't understand the need for planning. If countries don't plan properly, or donors don't understand how little infrastructure there is before they give the money, we'll always be running to catch up.

What is the best part?

It's fun when we get a new request. It's exciting to work with the country to define what they need and how we can handle it. I'm less interested in the process once something's up and running smoothly—I always want to move on to the next new thing! And although one can get a bit blasé about the size of the shipments, when we're sending out two jumbo jets full of medicine to help moms and kids—it's still a bit of a buzz.

What advice do you have for someone who is interested in your career?

Procurement is a huge part of the budget for any private company or government agency. That includes not just procuring goods but finding

Continued

consultants, offices spaces, and things the organization needs. Have a look at the supply chains for hospitals, look at the supply chain side of public health programs, and look at donor programs and at the services that help them. If you're interested in international work it helps to have overseas experience, even if it's short-term. Look for volunteer opportunities, and go even if it's just for a week or a month. The first overseas assignment is the toughest one to get, so don't wait around for a 3-year posting.

INTERNATIONAL PROGRAMS MANAGER

Job Description

The title "program manager" can have different meanings, but one typical role for a program manager at an international public health organization involves holding together various aspects of projects in the developing world. The job can include components of fundraising, grantmaking, logistics and planning, and technical advising. Often one manager handles multiple projects within a scope of work, such as HIV/AIDS prevention in an African country or region. In some cases, an organization collaborates with local, in-country NGOs that provide the staff to carry out the projects; in others, the program manager is managing work within his or her own organization. When a new program is being launched, the program manager guides the planning, making sure that projects and activities are based on sound science, are feasible and sustainable, and match the organization's and outside donors' goals. The program manager assists with development of the budget and may help write applications for funding. As the program gets underway, the program manager provides support to the staff, ensuring they have necessary supplies, training, transportation, and other needs. He or she tracks the progress of each project and makes sure that all work is in keeping with funders' rules and requirements. The program manager keeps funders, organization administrators, and others with a stake in the program informed about how the work is proceeding. Responsibilities also include communicating with other NGOs and with the country's Ministry of Health as needed to coordinate efforts, streamline the work, and ensure that local laws and regulations are followed. This job involves significant travel to project sites, often in areas with little development and few amenities.

Education and Certification

A typical requirement for a public health program manager is an MPH with a concentration in global health or a degree in international health or another related field. A bachelor's degree in a field such as public health is sometimes acceptable, with appropriate experience. Program managers usually have at least a few years of experience in roles related to program administration.

Core Competencies and Skills

- Love of travel and the ability to handle adverse conditions
- Familiarity with key public health issues and the ability to learn new information quickly
- Understanding of public health programs in both theory and practice
- Familiarity with local politics and culture
- Knowledge of rules and regulations that apply to funding from foundations and from the U.S. government
- Strong management skills, including organization, budgeting, and personnel management
- Ability to handle pressure and meet deadlines
- Excellent spoken and written communication skills

Compensation

Salaries increase with experience and responsibility; there is too much variation among jobs to give a single salary estimate. As a rough example, a starting salary at a nonprofit organization might be around $40,000, rising to $60,000 to $80,000 with experience.

Workplaces

Program managers doing international public health work are often found at nonprofit organizations and at consulting firms that contract with government and intergovernmental agencies.

Employment Outlook

Finding this type of work can take some determination. As with other global health jobs, good ways to get started include volunteering overseas, making connections, and being willing to accept a lower-level job and work your way up. Program manager can be a step along the way to a job with more responsibility and higher pay.

For Further Information

■ International Career Employment Weekly
www.internationaljobs.org

PUBLIC HEALTH PROFILE: International Programs Manager
April Davies, MPH
International Programs Manager
Water.org, Kansas City, MO

Describe the sort of work you do.

Water.org is a U.S.-based NGO that works with partner organizations in other countries to support water, sanitation, and hygiene projects. Water.org aims for a few specific elements in our projects. We like to see that women are involved, we like projects to be community driven, and we prefer to know that after the project is completed, the community will be able to sustain it. I'm the person who manages the projects, either working directly with our partner organizations or working with our country offices in Kenya and India. It's rare that I go long-term to our overseas offices, but I'll travel to our project countries for a week or two at a time.

What is a typical day like at your job?

My day at headquarters starts with conference calls in the early morning, because we have a 9-hour time difference with our partners in East Africa. Then I might work on reviewing project proposals or writing grant proposals. Sometimes I prepare information for our communications department to share with reporters, donors, or other nonprofits.

I often communicate with our partner organizations by email, too, answering questions and handling administrative issues. If the price of cement goes up, for example, they might want to know if they should ask for more funding or scale back their activities. I also hear from

Continued

other organizations in the regions we serve. A smaller NGO might be looking for a drilling rig, and they'll ask if one of our partners has one.

When I'm overseas, I meet with partner organizations and visit project sites. Some are in urban areas and some in remote locations. One project I've gone to see is in a very rural area of Ethiopia—you can't even travel to the communities during the rainy season. The communities have hand-dug shallow wells, and our partner organization goes out to cap each well and put a pump on it. For a sanitation project that involves building model latrines and then providing education so people can build their own, I'll talk with the educators and go out to see the latrines.

What education or training do you have? Is it typical for your job?

I have bachelor's degrees with majors in Spanish and journalism, and I have an MPH with a global health concentration and a community health and development focus. Water.org also employs engineers to tell us if projects are sound, and we have people who are experts in development and in micro-finance.

What path did you take to get to the job you are in today?

My first major international experience was the Peace Corps, right after college. I was assigned to a rural area in El Salvador. When I got there, the community had wells and a river but no water from a tap or a faucet. They wanted a water system that would be reliable and safe year round. I helped them get funding, purchase materials, and manage the finances. After the Peace Corps, I managed an AmeriCorps program that placed workers in safety-net clinics in underserved areas in Kansas. When I decided I wanted to go back to international health, I chose to earn an MPH at a school with good opportunities for field experiences. I got a work-study job with the school's water and sanitation group and stayed with them for a while after graduation, including spending 6 months in Kenya. I found my current job through an ad, but I'd been collaborating with Water.org on some projects already, so I was aware of them, and they were aware of me.

Continued

Where might you go from here, if you wanted to advance your career?

I've only been here for a short time, so I can see myself staying for a while. A more senior, supervisory position would be the next step, if I wanted to move straight up. Another option would be to move to an organization that hires people to manage work abroad, and to work in an office overseas.

What is the worst or most challenging part of your job?

I love having the opportunity to travel, but my colleagues and I don't like flying on small planes in other countries. It can be scary! In terms of the work itself, it's difficult when we have to disappoint our partner organizations, when we don't have the funding that they need to run at their ultimate capacity. Sometimes I see programs from other organizations that have good funding but aren't very effective or sustainable, and that can be frustrating.

What is the best part?

I'm working with organizations all over the world to solve water, sanitation, and hygiene challenges. I especially like the solutions our partners come up with, and I like sharing ideas with them. It's exciting to see that things work. It's also exciting to discover what doesn't work out that well and to take those lessons to create more solutions.

What advice do you have for someone who is interested in your career?

Gain international experience. Live and work in another country. And do it early on, because it's difficult to find organizations that will hire people to do international work if they haven't had international experience. Volunteering is one option, and study abroad doesn't hurt. Learning another language is also a good idea. Be flexible about the part of the world you go to. If it's in a country you weren't interested in, but it's a job you would like, go!

NGO FOUNDER/DIRECTOR

Job Description

"Nongovernmental organization" (NGO) is a term used to describe a broad range of organizations that provide services or work toward influencing public policy. NGOs are usually nonprofit organizations, although some are for-profit companies with strong public service orientations. Public health-oriented NGOs include large international foundations, tiny grassroots groups in developing countries, and everything in between. The director or president of a large NGO has responsibilities similar to those of the leader of any large organization. But running a small NGO in a developing country can be a different job entirely. These leaders are intimately involved in the day-to-day functions of the organization. Together with a small staff, they come up with ideas and do what's needed to get projects done. They track down potential funders, write grant proposals, plan events, meet with government officials, train staff members, and even take part in providing services.

When an American sets out to start or lead an NGO in a developing country, he or she is often coming in as an outsider, so one of the most important tasks is to gain the trust and cooperation of the local community. There's no point handing out mosquito nets if people have no intention of using them—or if they already have plenty. Long-term planning is another vital responsibility. If the NGO is digging wells to provide water, it is important not only to install pumps, but to provide for safety monitoring and maintenance. Many NGOs in developing countries hire primarily local citizens, who often have little experience creating or running social programs. Another of the NGO leader's tasks may be to train these local workers, with the goal of eventually giving them ownership of the organization.

Education and Certification

Educational requirements depend on the specific needs and purpose of the organization. Only people with demonstrated leadership skills and experience with the specific locations and programs will be hired to run established NGOs. Anyone can found an NGO, but only those with strong organizational and leadership skills will succeed. The skills and knowledge gained while earning an MPH can be very helpful, as can the experience of running a business or another nonprofit. Overseas experience is almost essential, because trying to get things done in a developing country can present challenges wildly different from anything Americans have experienced at home. A good way to get this experience is to begin with an entry-level job or even a volunteer position in an NGO whose goals match your passions.

Core Competencies and Skills

- Flexible thinking
- Adventurous spirit
- Optimism
- Persistence
- Exceptional managerial and financial skills
- Fluency in the local language (not always essential but very helpful)
- Thorough understanding of local culture and needs
- Excellent networking skills, with the ability to convince others to contribute funding, expertise, or time

Compensation

It's impossible to give a "typical" salary for the leader of an NGO focusing on public health issues overseas. Large organizations pay their executive directors handsomely, and they have staff members who work full time to bring in grants and donations. The leaders of small NGOs must raise the funds to pay their own and their employees' salaries. Compensation may reach the level of a modest salary by U.S. standards. If funding is tight, the leader of a new organization may even forgo payment while working to get the NGO off the ground.

Workplaces

NGOs exist in countries throughout the world. Depending on the size and structure of the organization, the job can mean living in a developing country or being based in the United States or another developed country and traveling to local sites as needed.

Employment Outlook

It is likely that there will always be a need for public health-oriented NGOs, because there will always be a need for improvement in public health infrastructure, services, and policy. There are organizations already in existence to meet many needs, and there are numerous opportunities to work at established NGOs and eventually achieve a leadership role. Those interested in starting new organizations should assess the need carefully, to avoid duplicating efforts already in progress.

For Further Information

■ Global Health Council
  www.globalhealth.org

PUBLIC HEALTH PROFILE: NGO Founder/Director
Asheesh Bhalla, MPH
President/Executive Director
The Friends of Humanity Organization of Afghanistan (FHO), Kabul, Afghanistan/Washington, D.C.

Describe the sort of work you do.

I direct a small NGO based in Afghanistan. Our goal is to strengthen the public health infrastructure of Afghanistan through the delivery of clinical treatment, public health education, and social development programs, with a focus on women. Women are key to Afghan society, but after 30 years of war, many have been left without resources. Their husbands may have died or been seriously injured, their extended families may have died, and many are caring for seven or eight children. And when the Taliban were in control, there wasn't much access to women's health care, so there isn't much infrastructure. The capacity just isn't there.

We run a 20-bed clinic in Kabul and a 30-bed clinic in Jalalabad. We do everything from check-ups to treating pneumonia to emergency deliveries. We have classrooms to train nurses and community health workers. We do seminars where our maternal health director teaches clients about nutrition, hygiene, what to expect during pregnancy. We're also doing a community dialogue program with women. We give them a safe space to talk about issues that concern them, such as religion or economics.

Continued

What is a typical day like at your job?

Developing a small organization in Afghanistan requires a lot of work in different areas. Right now, I'm based back in the United States, but until recently I was living full time in Afghanistan. On a typical day you might have found me collecting statistics, writing proposals, discussing partnerships, or looking at plans at a construction site. I'd start by checking my email. Then I'd talk with my colleagues about what we were working on, and I'd meet with the doctor at the clinic about what we needed. Sometimes I'd have a meeting with a government official or someone from another organization. When we were building the clinic, I'd visit the construction site. Some days I'd spend thinking about how to get past roadblocks, what to do if a funder changed their mind, or where to look for what we needed. We also have a program that provides vitamin A and antiparasite medication to children at orphanages, and some days I would go to help give these medicines.

What education or training do you have? Is it typical for your job?

I have a BA from an individualized study program. My concentration was political and economic trade policy and its effects on social development. I also hold an MPH with a concentration in health policy and management. There is no minimum education for a job like this, but I think that a strong education in public health is one of the best backgrounds you could have.

What path did you take to get to the job you are in today?

During college and graduate school, I worked on political campaigns, did an internship at the United Nations, and was a research assistant for Doctors without Borders. For my summer practicum for the MPH, I worked with an NGO affiliated with the best hospital in Afghanistan. I wrote hospital policy and did management training. I had all these great ideas from my public health training, but I found out that working in the real world is very different. Many of the things I tried to do failed! But what I learned, I was able to apply to starting a new NGO.

Continued

I came back to the U.S. and finished my MPH, but I wasn't interested in any jobs here. I tried to get a job with the U.S. government in Afghanistan, but I didn't have the right experience. I was asked to start the NGO by my two Afghan partners, whom I met while working in Afghanistan that first time.

Where might you go from here, if you wanted to advance your career?

Right now I'm attending law school while continuing to serve as executive director of FHO. I'm not sure what I'll do next. Starting a business in the health care sector is a possibility. I think with a couple more years experience, I could be hired to run another NGO, but I'm not sure I want to do that. I feel an attachment to the one I helped start.

What is the worst or most challenging part of your job?

Sometimes things take longer than you'd like. When we were building a clinic, I thought it would be finished by the end of June, but construction didn't finish until October!

What is the best part?

I get to brainstorm and plan projects and come up with programming ideas. So much is needed, and there are a lot of different things you can do. And our work environment in Afghanistan was so collegial. I was surrounded by people starting other NGOs, so we were bouncing ideas off each other and getting each others' perspective.

What advice do you have for someone who is interested in your career?

Stay hungry and stay foolish. I was told by plenty of people that I was crazy for going to Afghanistan and trying to work there, much less start an NGO. But when I first came to Afghanistan I was lucky to have a position that gave me so much responsibility and experience, and I used it to my advantage.

ENTOMOLOGIST

Job Description

Entomologists study bugs. That includes the insects that eat our crops and the honeybees that pollinate flowers. So what does this have to do with global health? Public health entomologists work with the insects that carry disease. Here in the United States, mosquitoes are mostly just a nuisance. But in many places in the world, mosquitoes carry malaria— one of the world's biggest killers. Dengue fever, another mosquito-borne infection, is a leading cause of childhood illness and death in some parts of Asia. Certain types of flies, ticks, fleas, and other insects can carry serious diseases, as well. There are public health entomologists studying these insects in laboratories, looking for ways to control their populations or reduce the risk of disease transmission. There are public health entomologists working in the field, doing surveillance of insect populations, studying local conditions, and helping to plan programs for insect control. This job can involve hands-on work examining sites and collecting samples; time in a lab or in front of a computer, pulling together data from multiple sources; and meetings, trainings, and presentations to share information with other public health professionals.

In addition to international jobs, there are entomologists working on insect control here in the United States, to protect us from infections like tick-borne Lyme disease and mosquito-borne West Nile virus. Public health entomologists also had a role in pest control after hurricane Katrina.

Education and Certification

Many jobs require a master's degree, and an entomologist usually needs a PhD to conduct independent research. A small number of universities offer bachelor's degrees in entomology; master's and PhD programs are more common. Entomologists can earn board certification from the Entomological Society of America.

Core Competencies and Skills

- Interest in problem-solving
- Passion for science
- Understanding of epidemiology
- Appreciation for local culture and an understanding of local practices
- Knowledge of the principles of vector control

- Ability to work with administrators and other nonscientists
- Relevant technical knowledge, such as how to use Geographic Information Systems (mapping systems to track disease)

Compensation

Salary will depend on the specific job and location. Income can range from the $20,000s for someone just starting out with a bachelor's degree to more than $100,000 for a PhD in a leadership role.

Workplaces

Public health entomologists are doing work related to international public health at universities, nonprofit organizations, government agencies, and consulting firms. Some entomologists work for the military, finding ways to protect soldiers from vector-borne diseases in locations throughout the world. There are even entomologists at for-profit companies developing products for insect control.

Employment Outlook

There are many job opportunities for entomologists, but the number of jobs in international public health is fairly small. Jobs in academia, where much of the international health research is carried out, can be very competitive.

For Further Information

- Entomological Society of America (ESA)
  www.entsoc.org
- CDC Division of Vector-Borne Infectious Diseases (DVBID)
  www.cdc.gov/ncidod/dvbid
- See also the organizations listed with disease ecologist.

REFERENCES

Fried, L. P., Bentley, M. E., Burke, D. S., Frenk, J. J., Klag, M. J., & Spencer, H. C. (2010). Global health is public health. *The Lancet, 375*, 535–537.

Koplan, J. P., Bond, C., Merson, M. H., Reddy, K. S., Rodriguez, M. R., Sewankambo, N. K., et al., Consortium of Universities for Global Health Executive Board. (2009). Towards a common definition of global health. *The Lancet, 373*, 1993–1995.

Off the Beaten Path

In the preceding chapters, you've learned about many traditional (and some nontraditional) careers in public health. This chapter is a mix of "everything else." Some of these jobs are likely to be part of the future of public health. Some are here because they're particularly exciting or fun. As you review these careers, keep in mind that public health is constantly changing and evolving. There is always room for new discoveries and new innovations.

For more ideas about emerging careers in public health, check out the course catalogs from some schools of public health—there are often classes that cover new developments and trends. And there are always interesting people to meet and careers to discover at APHA's annual meeting, where innovations from all areas of public health are presented and discussed.

DANCE INSTRUCTOR

Job Description

Maybe it's not fair to include dance instructor in a book about public health careers, because it's not something you'd find as a full-time job at the health department. But dance does have a role in public health.

We've learned that it's not enough just to tell people to go out and exercise, that it will improve health and fight diseases related to obesity—exercise has to be something they *want* to do. And we're all more likely to do things if they're fun. That's what's great about dance. A few years ago, more than 30 cities around the United States shared in a "Day of Dance" as part of a heart health campaign to help people see that getting fit can actually be fun. Many local health departments link citizens to dance classes at city recreation centers. Dance also turns up in campaigns focused on other issues—hip-hop dance and music being used as a medium to teach kids about health, for example.

Education and Certification

There is no single path to becoming a dance instructor. Some instructors learn at for-profit dancing schools. A degree (bachelor's, master's, or even a PhD) in dance or dance education is probably the best-respected credential. Public school dance teachers must have state certification to teach.

Core Competencies and Skills

- Excellent teaching skills
- Ability to inspire enthusiasm
- Patience with people who are not natural dancers
- Ability to design classes for specific needs
- Initiative to create new programs and seek funding to support them
- Knowledge of the evidence for a connection between dance and fitness—and the ability to explain it

Compensation

Instructors who teach "self enrichment" classes (classes that are essentially for fun, as opposed to professional training) earn a median salary of about $36,000, or an average of $20 per hour.

Workplaces

Dance instructors work at community centers, dance studios, schools, senior centers, daycare centers—anywhere there is room to dance and where people are interested in learning.

Employment Outlook

The future of dance in public health isn't clear. Combating obesity and sedentary lifestyles has been an increasingly strong focus of public health in recent years, and there is a need for new and creative programs with a basis in sound science. There are no guarantees, but learning what's known about the health benefits of dance and then networking with people from the local schools and health department could lead to interesting opportunities.

For Further Information

- American Alliance for Health, Physical Education, Recreation, and Dance (AAHPERD)
  www.aahperd.org
- Let's Move
  letsmove.gov

URBAN PLANNER

Job Description

Urban planner may not be "off the beaten path" of public health for long. Urban planners use computer programs and databases to collect and analyze information about population, transportation, and housing. They map out land areas and look at population density, demographics, roads and public transportation. They make recommendations for zoning, for the location of roads and schools, and for other aspects of city infrastructure, keeping local laws and regulations in mind. The job combines visits to development sites and time in the office, plus meetings with government officials and community groups.

Historically, urban planning and public health were closely connected. As sanitation improved, the two disciplines became disengaged. But with more and more attention to the impact that the environment has on people's health, there is a movement to bring urban planning and public health together. Public health professionals are asking whether neighborhoods can be built in a way that promotes diversity and reduces health disparities. They're looking at building safety into street designs, thinking about pedestrians and bicycles, not just cars. Some urban planners are already working on these types of issues—and if certain public health experts have their way, the future may see the two disciplines becoming integrated once again.

Education and Certification

A master's degree in urban or regional planning is required for most entry-level jobs. As of 2009, only two states required licensing or registration for urban planners. Professional certification, which can help with advancement, is available from the American Institute of Certified Planners. A few universities offer joint degrees in public health and urban planning.

Core Competencies and Skills

- Creativity
- Understanding of the intersection between the built environment and public health
- Ability to see how two-dimensional plans will translate into three-dimensional space
- Ability to both give and accept constructive criticism regarding plans
- Strong computer skills, including the ability to use geographic information systems

Compensation

In 2008, the median salary for urban and regional planners was about $60,000. Most earned between $37,000 and $92,000.

Workplaces

Most urban planners work for local governments. A few are at the CDC. Planners also work for private companies at architecture and engineering firms. Planners with a specific interest in public health can often be found at universities, doing research and teaching the next generation.

Employment Outlook

Employment growth is expected to be faster than average for this career, and the best opportunities will be in relatively wealthy communities with rapid growth. However, opportunities will also depend on city budgets and the state of the economy.

For Further Information

- American Planning Association (APA)
  www.planning.org

HOSPITAL ADMINISTRATOR

Job Description

Being the top administrator at a hospital isn't always a "public health" sort of job. The head of the hospital has to ensure that the place is profitable (or, for a nonprofit hospital, that income is meeting financial needs), in addition to keeping an eye on the services delivered and ensuring that the board of directors, medical staff, and department heads are all working toward the same goals. But some administrators make it their business to take a public health stance. Hospital administrators can spearhead quality improvement efforts. They can launch community health programs and support research into the community's needs. They can partner with local organizations and health departments to help meet current needs and prepare for future ones. And they can ensure that the hospital is prepared for epidemics and other potential crises. In addition to the top job, larger hospitals also have mid-level administrators who oversee various aspects of the hospital's services and behind-the-scenes management, and who report back to the top administrator. This is an office job with many meetings and obligations. Administrators also visit the various hospital departments so that they can see what is really happening in management and patient care.

Education and Certification

A typical way to prepare for a career as a hospital administrator is to earn a master's degree in health services administration, public administration, or business administration, and to start with a low-level administrative job at a hospital or health care center. More experience allows access to higher-level jobs with more responsibility. Some hospital administrators start out as physicians and gradually move from a clinical to an administrative role. Administrators who are members of the American College of Healthcare Executives (ACHE) can earn board certification and the title of ACHE Fellow by meeting certain professional requirements and passing an examination.

Core Competencies and Skills

- Strong leadership skills and the ability to inspire others
- Ability to handle multiple complex tasks
- Confidence in decision-making
- Good political and networking skills
- Significant administrative experience, including strategic planning and finance
- Understanding of the many needs within a hospital, from the cafeteria to the intensive care unit
- Understanding of the laws, regulations, and policies that apply to hospitals, from workforce issues to infection control

Compensation

At a large hospital network in a major city, the CEO can take home a base salary of more than half a million dollars each year, not counting bonuses and other benefits. Pay is lower at smaller hospitals. According to an IRS survey of nonprofit hospitals that began in 2006, the median salary for top administrators was $377,000. At small hospitals, the median salary was just $125,800, while at hospitals with annual revenues over $500 million, the median was $700,000.

Workplaces

Hospital administrators work for both for-profit and nonprofit hospitals. Some oversee networks including multiple hospitals and outpatient offices, while others are responsible for just one hospital.

Employment Outlook

There are plenty of lower-level administrative jobs, and the U.S. Bureau of Labor Services estimates that the job outlook for medical and health services managers will be good in the next few years, meaning that there will be about as many openings as there are people seeking these jobs. However, the top job of hospital president or CEO is extremely competitive, and only the best-qualified people will have a shot at these jobs.

For Further Information

- American College of Healthcare Executives (ACHE) *www.ache.org*

CHEF

Job Description

Not long ago, celebrity chef Jamie Oliver demonstrated how far our culture has gotten away from fresh, healthful food. He showed a group of American schoolchildren a tomato and asked them what it was. They didn't know. They couldn't name a cauliflower or an eggplant, either. There's been a lot of talk in public health about combating obesity by encouraging healthier eating, but if you just put an apple on a child's lunch tray, there's a good chance it's going to end up in the trash. You can offer adults all the fresh produce in the world—but if they don't know how to prepare it, they're not likely to choose fresh broccoli. A lot of people don't even know how to cook. And these days, many of us eat in front of the television, which can mean gulping down calories without noticing what we've eaten.

There is a small but dedicated movement among talented cooks to change all this. These chefs are showing people how to *enjoy* their fruits and veggies—how to make them a practical part of everyday meals that aren't just good for you, but absolutely delicious. Some chefs teach for love of food and the social sharing around the table; some are thinking of the environment; and some have health specifically in mind—but in each case, home cooking leads to healthier food choices. Chefs are helping revamp school meals, pushing to make cooking classes part of the school day, teaching parents and children to cook together, and running garden-to-table programs where kids grow their own produce and then learn to prepare it. Just like the dentists who come to our schools and teach our kids about oral hygiene, these chefs are giving kids the skills they need to make healthy habits part of their everyday lives.

Education and Certification

Chefs often have associate's or bachelor's degrees in culinary arts. There are also many chefs who learned their skills on the job.

Core Competencies and Skills

- Love of food
- Ability to create enthusiasm in others
- High level of comfort with public speaking
- At least a basic understanding of nutrition

- Strong teaching skills and the patience to teach people who know nothing about cooking
- Understanding of differences in people's food preferences, including cultural differences

Compensation

The median salary for a chef or head cook is about $39,000, with most earning $22,000 to $67,000. These numbers are for traditional chefs, though, who direct the cooking at restaurants and other food establishments. Some school cooking programs pay salaries in the $30,000 to $40,000 range, but it depends very much on the funding available.

Workplaces

Chefs who teach kids—or adults—to cook work primarily for nonprofit organizations.

Employment Outlook

The number of schools with cooking classes and gardens is small, but it's growing. Cooks who are interested can look for local programs or talk with school authorities, local foundations, or the health department about getting something started.

For Further Information

- Chez Panisse Foundation
  chezpanissefoundation.org
- Slow Food USA
  www.slowfoodusa.org

PUBLIC HEALTH PROFILE: Chef
Esther Cook

Chef Teacher
The Edible Schoolyard, a program of the Chez Panisse Foundation, Berkeley, CA

Continued

Describe the sort of work you do.

The Edible Schoolyard program provides gardening and cooking classes at a public school in Berkeley, California. The kids have garden classes through the science department and come to the kitchen through their history and humanities classes. We grow a wide variety of foods in the garden, so that the students can see what different crops look like. Hopefully, we're taking away the idea that good, fresh food is an elitist thing, and we're showing that everyone can have good food. The founder of the Edible Schoolyard, the chef Alice Waters, is committed to child nutrition as a basic right as well as an essential component of the learning process. She believes that mealtime, shared with family and friends, is an important ritual that teaches values and builds community. This tradition that is getting lost as fewer families eat together.

Part of my job is to illuminate for the kids that healthy is not synonymous with unpleasant. We don't focus on calories or a lot of nutritional information, because they're not there yet. Instead we seduce them with delicious food. For example we'll do an apple tasting. We'll try nine different apples, and they can see which ones they like.

What is a typical day like at your job?

My assistant and I teach two classes a day, sometimes three. We'll have all the food and vegetables laid out on the table and encourage students to use all of their senses as they cook their way through a lesson. We'll show them kale, and we'll talk about what it looks like and feels like. We'll show them neat things like how water beads up on the leaves when you rinse it, which elevates the experience from simply washing food to observing how beautiful an ordinary task can be.

After the kids do all the prep and the cooking, then we'll clear the table and set it with a tablecloth. We sit down together, and we eat together. For some kids, that's their only experience of eating together—their families don't do this. They learn how to have a conversation at the table and how to pass food, and in the process they gain a sense of accomplishment and pride. The kids do the clean-up, too.

In addition to the class time, I also go shopping at farmers' markets, because not everything we use comes from our garden. There's lesson planning and research. We've written manuals, and we do

Continued

what we call academies for educators who want to start programs like ours. We also have staff meetings, we have visitors, and there is a fair amount of media attention.

What education or training do you have? Is it typical for your job?

I don't know what's typical, because not a lot of people have my job. Hopefully it's becoming more common, though. There are a lot of cooking programs you can go to if you want to learn to be a chef, but I just worked in restaurants and learned that way. Because the Edible Schoolyard is a nonprofit program, I don't have to be a certified teacher. A certified teacher does have to be present, though.

What path did you take to get to the job you are in today?

I went to college for fine arts and I've taken classes in child development. I ended up as a cook because for me it was a way to continue to do art, but still earn money. I started volunteering for the Center for Urban Education about Sustainable Agriculture. We would go into schools and do little cooking projects, with desks pushed together and no running water. And the kids would get so fired up—it was great to see that!

A friend told me about the chef teacher job. I'd been running a similar program in a community center, but it was only for 6 weeks at a time. I hadn't known about the Edible Schoolyard program, but I knew who Alice Waters was. And my parents were teachers, so even though I'd never been a teacher, I understood about teaching and really appreciated it. I got the job, and I became a founding teacher here. It's been 13 years, and I've never looked back!

Where might you go from here, if you wanted to advance your career?

I joke that they're going to have to blast me out of here eventually, because I'm not leaving. I've always been fascinated by the therapeutic aspects of cooking, though, and I'd like to look into cooking in the same way that art therapy came about. There are some troubled kids

Continued

at the school, and I've been really moved by the transformations that you see in them when they're in the kitchen.

What is the worst or most challenging part of your job?

Sometimes it's just hard to see other people's realities. To realize that not every child is getting this experience. As wonderful as it is to have the Edible Schoolyard, it should be a part of every school.

What is the best part?

Absolutely, without a doubt, the kids are the best part. Getting to be a part of their lives on a daily basis gives me so much optimism for the future. They are so bright and so funny and so insightful.

What advice do you have for someone who is interested in your career?

Volunteer! We've had so many volunteers move on to paid positions. Look at places you admire and offer to help them for a few months, and see if you like it. And if the program you are interested in does not have an opening, look for other programs that might.

WORKSITE WELLNESS MANAGER

Job Description

Health and wellness programs have shown up in corporate settings across the United States. Employers like them because they have the potential to reduce health insurance costs and boost productivity. The motive is often profit—but one result, if it's done right, is better health for employees. The person responsible for corporate wellness designs programs and policies (or purchases services from outside vendors) to encourage employees to quit smoking, exercise more, eat better, cope with stress more effectively, and generally make better choices for their health. Ideally, these are evidence-based efforts with a focus on concrete results. The wellness manager collects information about health challenges common among employees and about employees' interests. The manager devises interventions based on that information, then collects more data once the interventions are underway to be sure they are working. An important goal is to make the work environment conducive to health. Examples of interventions include posting calorie information in the cafeteria, creating special discounts on healthier lunches, and working with vending machine suppliers to include more healthful snacks. A wellness program could offer flexible work hours to decrease employee stress levels. Some include financial incentives for employees who participate in weight management programs, keep their cholesterol under control, or try to quit smoking. If employees are interested, the wellness manager might even distribute pedometers to all employees and hold a walking contest, with prizes for the team that walks the most each week.

Education and Certification

Employers usually look for a bachelor's or master's degree in a field related to health promotion or exercise science; some ask for an MPH. Managing a program usually requires some experience in this field. Wellness practitioners can complete training programs through the Wellness Council of America (WELCOA) to earn certification as WELCOA Well Workplace practitioners.

Core Competencies and Skills

- Creativity to keep wellness programs fresh, even if the issues do not change
- Patience for employees who may start wellness activities but not finish them
- Good skills in persuasion and negotiation, for working with administrative staff to implement changes
- Knowledge of basic survey techniques and statistical methods
- Knowledge of how to translate research into practice and design evidence-based programs
- Understanding of outcomes assessment and quality improvement methods
- Understanding of social marketing

Compensation

The Wellness Professionals' Salary and Benefits Survey, published by the Wellness Program Management Advisor, found a range of salaries in

2007 to 2008. The average salary for a "wellness manager" was $69,500 and for a "wellness coordinator," $43,482.

Workplaces

There are worksite wellness programs at all types of organizations, including for-profit companies, nonprofits, and government agencies. Wellness managers also work for outside agencies and consulting firms that provide wellness services, and for insurance agencies.

Employment Outlook

Worksite wellness is a rapidly growing industry. In 2008, 54% of public sector full-time workers and 28% of private sector full-time workers had access to wellness programs, a substantial increase over the past decade. Future demand for wellness managers will be influenced by developments in health care reform and by the results of research on the effectiveness of wellness programs as money-saving efforts.

For Further Information

- Wellness Council of America (WELCOA)
  www.welcoa.org

MEDICAL EXPERT/MEDIA

Job Description

When President Obama floated the idea of television celebrity doctor Sanjay Gupta as Surgeon General, a lot of public health doctors were outraged. Dr. Gupta is a neurosurgeon and a journalist—not a public health expert. But the President did have a point. A doctor with a strong presence in the media can have a huge impact on how we think about health and on the choices we make. An awful lot of people got answers to questions about the flu pandemic from Dr. Gupta's broadcasts. Fans tune in each weekday to a health information show hosted by Dr. Mehmet Oz. People listen to the local doctor who does the "medical minute" on the evening news, too. There are also doctors working behind the scenes, advising movie and television scriptwriters, trying to keep drama from trumping accuracy, and sometimes even sneaking public health messages into the story. There are doctors helping with nonfiction television shows, ensuring that weight loss advice or a story about the latest way to prevent a heart attack is actually correct. Some doctors advise on social marketing efforts or write magazine and web articles about health and prevention. And we know that media can have an impact. Studies have shown that teens picked up messages about condoms from a television sitcom and that viewers remembered advice about cancer prevention from storylines on favorite dramas. And of course, the media is a major source of information whenever there is an immediate public health concern.

Education and Certification

A clinical degree is essential for credibility. Media advisors on medical issues are typically doctors, but nurses and nutritionists can have a role here, too. For doctors, having completed a clinical residency and being licensed is usually expected if not absolutely required.

Core Competencies and Skills

- Creativity
- Excellent networking skills
- Knack for translating medical information into plain language
- Good sense of what will hold the public's interest
- Awareness of how the general public uses and reacts to health information
- Media skills—not just public speaking skills, but an understanding of what works on camera
- Understanding of how media works, including video production, web design, and publishing

Compensation

A top "media doctor" with national exposure can earn far more than he would in private practice. Dr. Gupta would have taken a substantial pay cut if he had accepted the job as Surgeon General! Working in the media doesn't guarantee a fabulous salary, though. It very much depends on the job, the hours, and the audience reach. A reporter or freelance writer won't necessarily be paid extra just because he or she is an MD.

Workplaces

A doctor working in media could be a freelance writer or consultant, or an employee at a production company or television network. Some doctors collaborate with scriptwriters and producers part time, while maintaining a clinical practice or working as a professor at a medical school.

Employment Outlook

A lot of doctors want to do this kind of work, and there are only a handful of jobs—most of which are never advertised. That doesn't mean it can't happen. But it can take a lot creativity and perseverance, not to mention being in the right place at the right time.

For Further Information

■ National Association of Medical Communicators (NAMC)
www.namc.info

PUBLIC HEALTH PROFILE: Medical Expert
John Whyte, MD, MPH
Chief Medical Expert, Vice President of CME
Discovery Channel, Silver Spring, MD

Describe the sort of work you do.

My job at Discovery Channel is to create medical education and patient education programming. My department makes television shows that appeal to a physician audience as well as a lay audience, and we create media for Discovery's digital properties, too—Web sites, online games, podcasts, and streaming video. Discovery's strength is the power of storytelling, and everything we do is consistent with the theme of "Entertain your Brain." So a big part of my job is trying to reach a balance between giving quality, credible information, and providing entertainment. You can have the best health message out there, but if no one's listening it doesn't matter.

Continued

What is a typical day like at your job?

My day is split among working on new proposals for shows, helping to oversee production and editorial content, and managing the health aspects of our digital properties. I also have to stay current with the medical literature, so I read medical journals and articles from clipping services.

When we're planning our medical education shows, the first thing we do is figure out where physicians are not doing a good enough job in caring for their patients. What do they need to know? We also ask where patients need help in improving their own care. Then we look at potential funders, like pharmaceutical companies and large foundations, to see what they might be willing to sponsor. I work with members of my team as well as outside contractors to create grant proposals, and I look over the proposals before they go out to make sure they are medically accurate.

Our production team doesn't have medical knowledge, so I educate them about each show's topic. I contact outside experts to invite them to participate in the programs, and I approve the subjects for documentary-style segments. As the show is being produced, I review the video and give comments.

I'm the only physician at Discovery, so producers from other departments come to me for medical information, too. For Discovery's National Body Challenge, I make sure the experts they plan to use are qualified, and I give input on the fitness and weight loss recommendations. I also do a lot of digital video shorts, where I'm actually the one on camera. For a recent one, I went out onto the street and talked with people about aging and health.

What education or training do you have? Is it typical for your job?

I have an MD and an MPH, and I'm board-certified in internal medicine. I think in media, especially if you want to be on television, it helps to be board-certified in a specialty. People really equate that with quality. I also think having done a full clinical residency helps my work here. If you want to impact patients' behavior or physicians' practices, you have to understand how patients think, and you have

Continued

to understand the process of medicine. I still do some direct patient care, and that adds tremendous value.

What path did you take to get to the job you are in today?

I never expected to be working in media. I thought I would be a faculty member at a medical school, and eventually a department chair. But even in college, I was interested in health policy. During medical school, I took time out after my second year to earn an MPH. After my internal medicine residency, I did a heath services research fellowship, and I enjoyed that a lot. And then I had to figure out how to combine policy and clinical practice. I had some contacts in government who knew about my interests, so I reached out to them. It turned out they wanted to bring more physicians into Medicare policy work, and they created a spot for me. I really had to go out and make that opportunity, though. After that, I worked on childhood obesity issues at AHRQ. That job included working with the media, which is how I met the people at Discovery. At first, I wasn't interested in taking this job. But then I started thinking about how I could use the position to translate medical research into actual practice. Discovery is truly a global multimedia company, with many opportunities to have an impact.

Where might you go from here, if you wanted to advance your career?

I want to find even more effective ways to change behavior and to communicate health messages. This is complex information, and people often don't want to hear it. They don't want to be preached to. I don't necessarily have another job in mind, but I'm always interested in opportunities to learn to communicate health message better.

What is the worst or most challenging part of your job?

I may have a great idea for a show, but I need to find the funding. That can be very challenging, especially in a tough economic climate. And we have to keep seeking funding constantly for all our shows—it can be exhausting!

Continued

Traveling does get tiresome after a while, too. I spend a lot of time in airports and trains, when I could be attending to other priorities. But what's cool is that our shows have taken me to every continent except Antarctica.

What is the best part?

The best part of the job is having the ability to create a show on a health topic where I know there needs to be improvement. I can wake up one day and say, "I really want to educate people about taking better care of type 2 diabetes." And I can go out and obtain funding and make a program that will be seen by millions of people.

It's also exciting, here at Discovery Channel, to be surrounded by some of the most creative people around. You don't usually get that when you're practicing medicine.

What advice do you have for someone who is interested in your career?

I would say to get a good education, to have good clinical knowledge so that you can be a medical advisor. You also need to be willing to network and to develop a group of people who know and respect you. Often you can reach out to people who have careers similar to what you would like to do and ask them about their career path and how they got involved. Some of the best career opportunities are not listed in any job description. You have to create them.

The Future of Public Health

PART III

23 The Future of Public Health

HEALTH REFORM AND PUBLIC HEALTH JOBS

After reading all the "employment outlook" segments in this book, you may be feeling a little frustrated—because for so many of jobs profiled here, the answer to the question, "Will I find steady employment?" isn't clear. As a matter of fact, among the hundred or so people who contributed information to this book, the most common answer to questions about job outlook was, "It depends."

As of this writing, a bill to reform the U.S. health care system has just been signed by the President. The bill promises to expand and improve health insurance coverage, providing access to care for many more Americans. There is another element of the bill that's getting less attention in the news, but that has public health professionals watching closely: an increase in funding for public health and prevention.

Why does this matter for public health careers? Right now, there are shortages in many areas of the public health workforce. In 2007, state health departments reported a severe shortage of public health nurses, and many states had shortages of epidemiologists, laboratorians, and environmental health workers. Some places also lacked enough nutritionists, public health physicians, and social workers. But at the same time, health department budgets are being cut, and when people retire or move to other jobs the vacancies aren't necessarily being filled. Increased funding could mean a scale-up of surveillance and prevention programs, more job openings, and demand for a substantial number of well-trained public health professionals. Exactly what will happen remains to be seen, of course, but many public health professionals are hoping that health care reform will drive new attention to public health.

CLIMATE CHANGE AND PUBLIC HEALTH

There are already public health experts working at the intersection of climate change and public health. (Disease ecologists, entomologists, and community activists are just a few.) If projections about climate change are correct, we may see significant changes not only in weather, but in patterns of disease—and we may need more public health professionals to combat these effects.

Many infectious diseases are strongly influenced by climate. According to the World Health Organization, climate change can alter both the geographic range and the transmission seasons of insect-borne diseases like malaria. Research suggests that with climate change, dengue fever could reach an extra two billion people by the 2080s.

Changes in rainfall can influence the supply of drinking water, too, through droughts or floods. Contaminated water can, in turn, lead to increases in diarrheal disease, which is responsible for over two million deaths each year, mainly in the developing world. Climate change can also disrupt agricultural rhythms, if drought or excess rainfall interferes with a season's crops. The collapse of agriculture in a region can lead to widespread malnutrition and a range of associated health problems. It can also lead to problems with sanitation and disease transmission, particularly if people must leave villages for crowded camps or big-city slums.

Preparedness is already a hot topic in public health, and the need for public health professionals who understand how to help in the wake of natural disasters may continue to expand. Since the 1960s, the number of weather-related disasters around the world has more than tripled. Developing countries are hardest hit, but we saw with hurricane Katrina that public health disasters can happen after natural disasters here at home, too.

Climate change can also affect air pollution, with higher temperatures raising the levels of pollutants. Studies have shown that deaths from heart disease go up in parallel with certain types of air pollution, and prolonged exposure may decrease life expectancy. Increased pollution and higher pollen levels can also exacerbate respiratory diseases like asthma.

PUBLIC HEALTH AND CHANGING POPULATIONS

Changes in populations, including population density, age distribution, and wealth all have significant impacts on people's health. In the developing world, migrations from rural to urban areas lead to changes in disease distribution, new sanitation issues, and new challenges to mental health. Even improvements in health care can create new challenges, such as a decrease in infant mortality leading to larger families with more mouths to feed.

Here in the United States, immigration patterns are also changing public health needs. An influx of new immigrants to a city can mean an increase in the ratio of children to adults, requiring the health department to shift funds and focus to meet different needs. People from different places may have different disease risks; hepatitis B, for example, is much more prevalent among immigrants from certain places than among the U.S. population as a whole, due to differing patterns of transmission. In places where the population is aging, a greater focus on elder health issues may be needed.

Funding for public health doesn't always parallel population needs, and it can be slow to catch up. But keeping an eye on shifts in local demographics, in the U.S. population, and in populations in other regions or nations can be helpful in predicting where new public health efforts will be needed.

NEW MEDIA AND PUBLIC HEALTH

There is promising new work in disease prevention and health promotion based on social media. During the 2009 to 2010 flu season, the CDC used Web site buttons, Twitter updates, a Facebook site, a Web site optimized for mobile phones, online videos, and a text messaging system to keep people informed about flu symptoms, treatment, and prevention, and about new developments. They also created a series of widgets, computer programs that could be embedded in web pages and updated automatically as new information emerged.

There are many other uses for new media in public health. Texts can be sent out to cell phones citywide, letting citizens know about weather emergencies, temporary boil alerts (when water may be contaminated and must be boiled before drinking), disease outbreaks, and other important happenings. Texts are being incorporated into emergency preparedness plans. Programs to promote prenatal care are using text messaging to send women information about pregnancy.

When peanut-containing products were recalled in 2009 due to concerns about salmonella contamination, the CDC created an online database of recalled products and a widget to help direct consumers to the site. Web sites such as flu.gov, AIDS.gov, and HealthierUS.gov give consumers quick access to health information and guidance about prevention. Public health agencies and organizations have tried using various forms of new media to reach populations that standard public health efforts miss.

Some of these efforts have been successful. Some have been less so—in part because public health professionals aren't always in tune with the latest fads. It's not clear whether new media will create a wave of new jobs in public health, but there is definitely a need for people who understand the Internet, social networking, and other forms of new media, and who can make them work for the cause of population-level health.

REFERENCES

World Health Organization. (January, 2010). *Climate change and health fact sheet.* Retrieved from http://www.who.int/mediacentre/factsheets/fs266/en/index.html
Reichardt, A., & Lewis, M. (2007). *2007 state public health workforce survey results.* Arlington, VA: Association of State and Territorial Health Officials.

Index